Book 2

MRCP 2

Practice Questions & Answers

Dermatology, Endocrinology and Metabolism,
Gastroenterology, Psychiatry,
and Renal Medicine

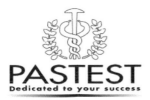

PASTEST
Dedicated to your success

Book 2

MRCP 2

Practice Questions & Answers

**Dermatology, Endocrinology and Metabolism,
Gastroenterology, Psychiatry,
and Renal Medicine**

Edited by

Philip Kelly
Department of Diabetes and Metabolism
Royal London Hospital
London

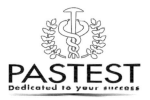

PASTEST
Dedicated to your success

© 2005 PASTEST Ltd
Egerton Court
Parkgate Estate
Knutsford
Cheshire
WA16 8DX

Telephone: 01565 752000

First published 2005

ISBN: 1 904627 26 9

A catalogue record for this book is available from the British Library.

PasTest Revision Books and Intensive Courses

PasTest has been established in the field of postgraduate medical education since 1972, providing revision books and intensive study courses for doctors preparing for their professional examinations. Books and courses are available for the following specialties:

MRCGP, MRCP Part 1 and 2, MRCPCH Part 1 and 2, MRCPsych, MRCS, MRCOG, DRCOG, DCH, FRCA, PLAB.

For further details contact:

PasTest, Freepost, Knutsford, Cheshire WA16 7BR
Tel: 01565 752000 Fax: 01565 650264
www.pastest.co.uk   enquiries@pastest.co.uk

Text prepared by Vision Typesetting Ltd, Manchester
Printed and bound by Cambrian Printers, Aberystwyth

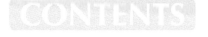

CONTENTS

Dermatology
Virginia Hubbard MBBS MRCP
Consultant Dermatologist, The Whittington Hospital, London.

Endocrinology and Metabolism
Philip Kelly MBBS MRCP
Department of Diabetes and Metabolism, Royal London Hospital,
London.

Gastroenterology
Peter Irving MA MRCP
Specialist Registrar in Gastroenterology, Whipps Cross University
Hospital, London.

Psychiatry
Neil Harrison MRCP MRCPsych
Clinical Research Fellow, Institute of Cognitive Neuroscience and
Honorary Specialist Registrar, Neuropsychiatry, National Hospital,
Queen Square.

Renal Medicine
Ravi Rajakaria BSc(Hons) MBChB MRCP
Experimental Medicine and Nephrology, William Harvey Research
Institute, London.

ACKNOWLEDGEMENTS

I would like to express my gratitude to the team at PasTest particularly Amy Smith and Cathy Dickens for their unswerving support and tolerance during the preparation of this book and series. Many patients have been gracious enough to contribute to our ongoing education by allowing their images to be used in these volumes. The series would have been impossible without the help of the following: Dr Ed Seward, The Middlesex Hospital, London for his comments on the gastroenterology chapter; Drs. S Whitely, N Power and O Chan, Radiology; Dr R Feakins, Pathology; Dr R Marley, Hepatology, Barts and The London NHS Trust; Dr R Makins, Homerton University Hospital NHS Trust and Dr J Mawdsley, Barts and The London, Queen Mary School of Medicine and Dentistry; Medical Photography, Radiology and Medicine, King George Hospital, Ilford; Medical Illustration at Barts and The London School of Medicine and Dentistry and The Department of Diabetes and Metabolism at The Royal London Hospital. Special thanks are due to Dr Alexandra Nanzer for her considered and helpful criticisms and delightful encouragement.

Philip Kelly

The MRCP (UK) Part 2 written examination consists of two 3-hour papers, each with up to 100 multiple choice questions; they are either one from five (best of 5) or 'n' from many, where two answers are chosen from ten. Each question will have a clinical scenario and might contain investigations to interpret; many might also contain an image. There is a pass-mark agreed by the examiners but a candidate's performance is also assessed in relation to other candidates.

This three-book series provides practice questions with extensive explanations to aid candidates preparing for the examination. The authors are all clinicians writing sections in their chosen fields and as such have been chosen for their clear understanding of the required knowledge base for this important exam. The breadth of knowledge for this exam is vast and they have attempted to cover the 'syllabus' as completely as possible. Great care has been taken to explain areas that cause difficulty as thoroughly as possible. No apology is made where the format of the questions differs slightly from the exam. These books are not merely practice papers but educational aids and where a topic can be best explained by diversion from the strict format of the exam, for the sake of understanding, this has been done.

This book covers dermatology, endocrinology and metabolism, gastroenterology, psychiatry, and renal medicine and is best taken – in concert with its partners within the series – as a supplement to a thorough clinical grounding, the general medical texts and the core clinical journals.

Any comments or suggestions on this book or the series will be gratefully received.

Chapter One

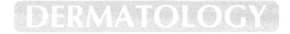

Case 1

A 42-year-old woman presented with a 6-month history of this appearance:

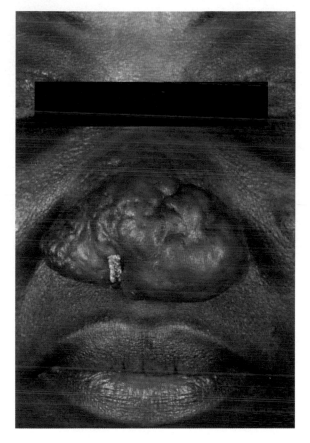

1   Which of the following would not be associated with this appearance?

- ☑ A   Radiolucent bone cysts on a plain X-ray of the hands
- ☐ B   Hypocalcaemia
- ☐ C   Symmetrical polyarthropathy involving the small joints of the hands
- ☐ D   Mikulicz syndrome
- ☐ E   Restrictive pattern on pulmonary function tests

Case 2

This 32-year-old woman presented with hair loss for 8 months.

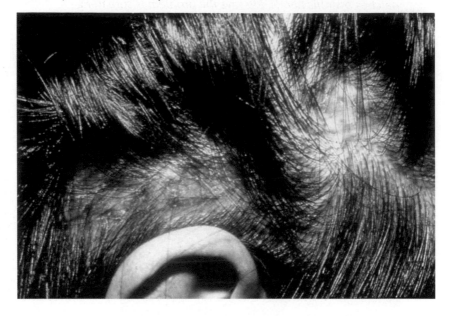

1   Which of the following would typically cause this pattern of hair loss?

- [ ] A   Discoid lupus erythematosus
- [ ] B   Dissecting cellulitis of the scalp
- [ ] C   Tinea capitis
- [ ] D   Hypothyroidism
- [x] E   Alopecia areata

Case 3

A 34-year old man presented with a 3-month history of depigmented patches over his hands. He says the problem is spreading

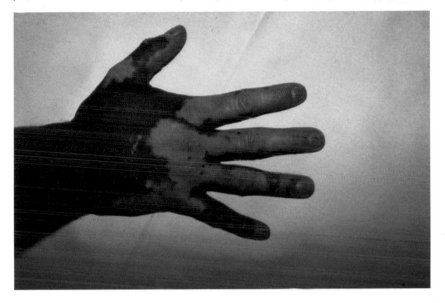

I   **Which of the following conditions has an increased incidence in association with this picture?**

☐   A   Lichen planus
☐   B   Hyperparathyroidism
☐   C   Sarcoidosis
☑   D   Pernicious anaemia
☐   E   Haemochromatosis

Case 4

This 67-year-old man with hypertension and epilepsy developed this rash while on holiday in southern Spain.

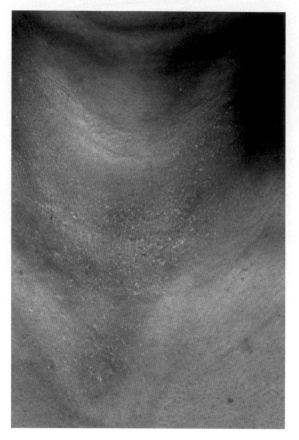

1   Which of his drugs is the most likely culprit in this pattern of drug rash?

☐ A   Atenolol
☐ B   Bendroflumethiazide
☐ C   Codeine phosphate
☑ D   Phenytoin
☐ E   Aspirin

Case 5

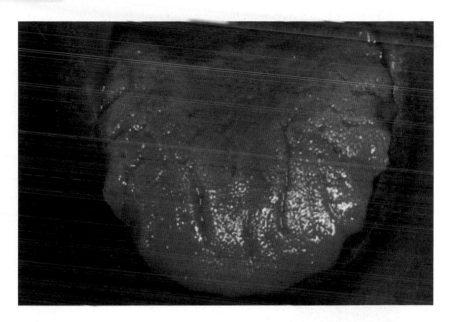

1 **Which of the following is not associated with the appearance of this tongue?**

- [ ] A Phenytoin treatment
- [ ] B Trisomy 21
- [ ] C Crohn's disease
- [ ] D Sarcoid
- [ ] E Geographical tongue

Case 6

A 31-year-old man returned from a holiday in Florida with this rash on his right shin. The rash spread at a rate of approximately 1 cm per day. He was systemically well.

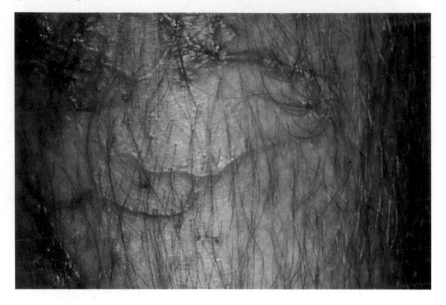

1   What is the likeliest pathogenic organism?

☐ A   *Toxocara canis*
☑ B   *Schistosoma haematobium*
☐ C   *Strongyloides stercoralis*
☐ D   *Sarcoptes scabei*
☐ E   *Ankylostoma braziliense*

Case 7

This 42-year old woman presented with excess facial hair.

1 Which of the following is not a recognised cause of this appearance?

☑ A   Spironolactone
☐ B   Congenital adrenal hyperplasia (CAH)
☐ C   Polycystic ovary syndrome (PCOS)
☐ D   Cushing's disease
☐ E   Hyperprolactinaemia

Case 8

A 38-year-old woman presented with a 6-month history of this appearance in both axillae. Her BMI was 35.

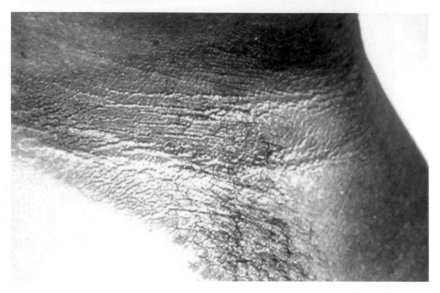

1   What is the most appropriate first investigation?

☑ A   Fasting glucose
☐ B   CXR
☐ C   Skin biopsy
☐ D   Ovarian ultrasound
☐ E   Colonoscopy

Case 9

A 78-year-old woman presents short of breath, with haemoptysis.

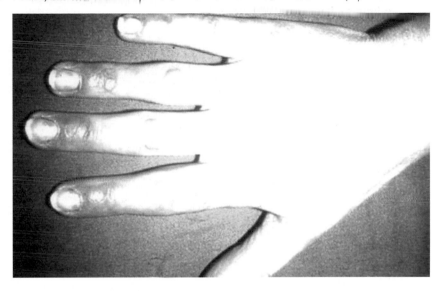

1 **What is the diagnosis?**

- [ ] A Lichen planus
- [ ] B Dermatomyositis
- [ ] C SLE
- [ ] D Psoriasis
- [ ] E Allergic contact dermatitis

Case 10

A 31-year-old man with ulcerative colitis had a laparotomy. Three weeks later the scar broke down, leaving this picture. Microbiology swabs were negative.

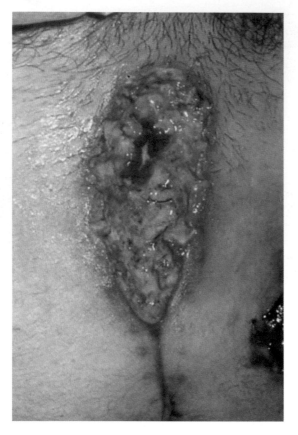

1   What is the most appropriate treatment for this?

- [ ] A   Broad-spectrum intravascular antibiotics
- [x] B   Surgical debridement
- [ ] C   Pulsed intravenous methylprednisolone
- [ ] D   Sulfasalazine
- [ ] E   Intravenous aciclovir

Case 11

A 31-year-old engineer returned from a trip to Saudi Arabia 2 months previously. He presented with a red nodule which subsequently ulcerated to give this appearance:

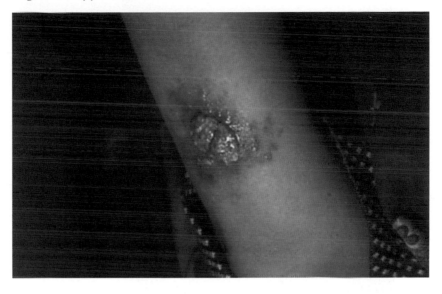

1   What is the most likely diagnosis?

☐   A   Mosquito bite
☐   B   Mycetoma
☐   C   Lepromatous leprosy
☑   D   Cutaneous leishmaniasis
☐   E   Lupus vulgaris

Case 12

A 38-year-old intravenous drug user presented with a 6-month history of an itchy rash over his wrists and ankles. He was hepatitis C-positive.

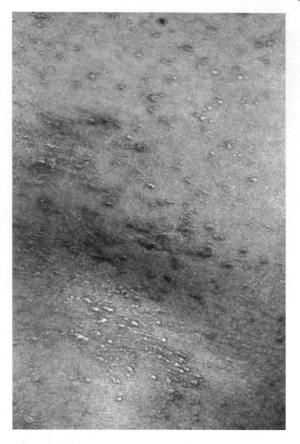

1   What is this rash?

☐   A   Eczema
☐   B   Scabies
☐   C   Psoriasis
☐   D   Secondary syphilis
☑   E   Lichen planus

Case 13

A 29-year-old man from Nigeria was admitted to hospital while visiting relatives in the UK, with a weak right hand. He was also noted to have this rash.

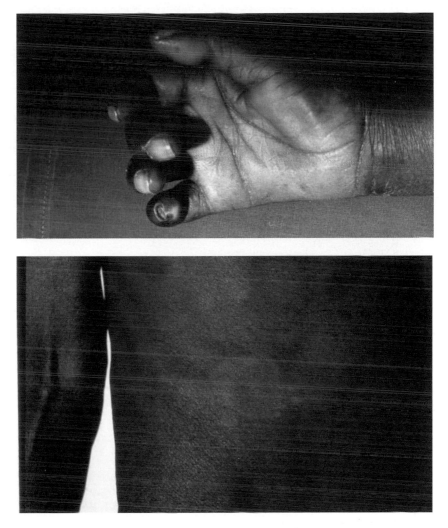

1   What is the unifying diagnosis?

☐   A   Vitiligo
☐   B   Psoriasis
☑   C   Granuloma annulare
☐   D   Leprosy
☐   E   Tuberculosis

Case 14

A 34-year-old woman was referred from the Psychiatric Unit with a 3-week history of a rash. This had started as widespread erythematous macules, but evolved to the picture below. She had commenced carbamazepine 1 month previously. She also had a urinary tract infection and had been started on co-trimoxazole earlier in the week.

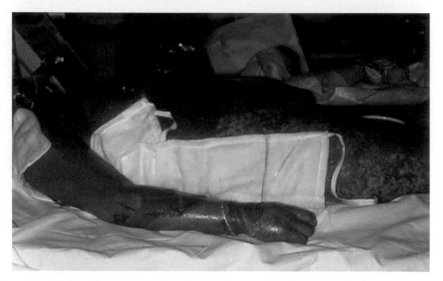

1 What is the most important therapeutic intervention?

- ☐ A Aggressive intravascular antibiotic treatment for urinary sepsis
- ☐ B Systemic corticosteroids
- ☑ C Withdraw carbamazepine
- ☐ D Insertion of a central venous line
- ☐ E Cool the body

Case 15

A 54-year-old woman presented with weight loss. These are her hands. She was ANA-negative.

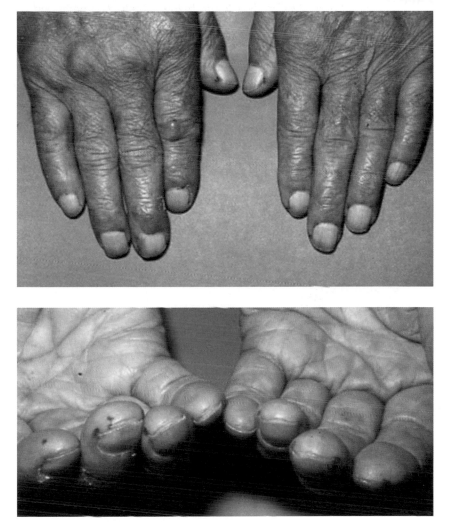

1   What is the diagnosis?

- A   Osteoarthritis
- B   Rheumatoid arthritis
- C   Pseudogout
- D   Systemic sclerosis
- E   SLE

Chapter Two

ENDOCRINOLOGY and METABOLISM

Case 1

A lady is followed up in the clinic with hypothyroidism. Her thyroid replacement is being titrated and she is currently taking 50 micrograms thyroxine once dialy.

On examination she is 85 kg, 1.65 m and the skin is cool and dry. The pulse is regular, low-volume and 52 bpm, JVP 4 cm, there is no oedema. The praecordium and lungs are normal. In the abdomen there is 2-cm hepatomegaly.

The following fasting investigations were performed before clinic:

Plasma glucose	6.0 mmol/L	random 7/1.1
Cholesterol	13.0 mmol/L	
HDL cholesterol	0.8 mmol/L	fasting 17
LDL cholesterol	1.9 mmol/L	
Triglycerides	7.3 mmol/L	2h 7.11.1

On her palms the following appearance is observed:

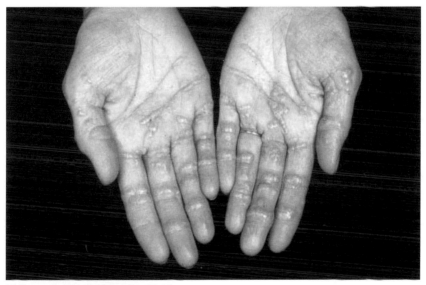

Wellcome Trust Medical Photographic Library

1 Which is the most likely diagnosis?

- [ ] A Hyperlipidaemia of diabetes
- [x] B Familial hypercholesterolaemia (type IIa hyperlipidaemia)
- [ ] C Familial combined hyperlipidaemia (type IIb hyperlipidaemia)
- [ ] D Familial hypertriglyceridaemia (type V hyperlipidaemia)
- [ ] E Familial dysbetalipoproteinaemia (type III hyperlipidaemia)

21

Case 2

You are referred a lady with thyrotoxicosis and exophthalmos. She has a moderate sized nodular goitre. The GP has already started her on carbimazole and this is her thyroid function while taking 5 mg once daily.

Free T$_4$	15.1 pmol/L
TSH	2.1 mU/L
Urine β-HCG	Negative

She has a neck scan and a CT orbit to assess the exophthalmos:

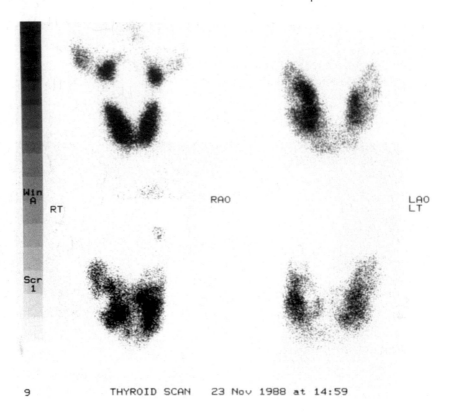

THYROID SCAN   23 Nov 1988 at 14:59

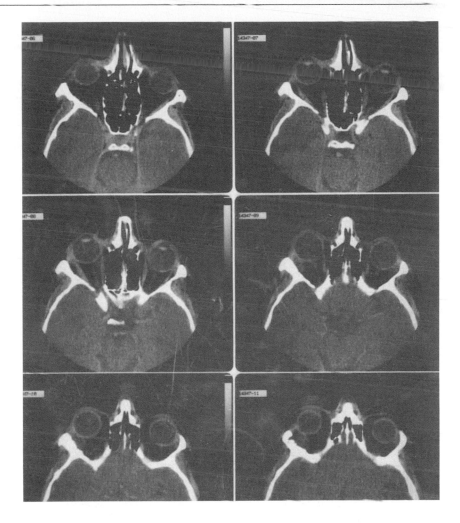

1 What is the next step?

- [ ] A Continue carbimazole, titrating the dose to suppress the TSI I to below the normal range
- [ ] B Prednisolone 0.5–1 mg per kg initially for 2–6 weeks
- [ ] C Referral to an ophthalmic surgeon
- [ ] D Referral to a radiotherapist to consider low-dose lens-sparing orbital radiotherapy
- [x] E Continue the current medication and consider radioiodine if the goitre becomes troublesome

Case 3

A 27-year-old man is referred with polyuria and thirst. He is on no medications; there is no family history. Weight 83 kg, height 1.92 m. His 24-hour urine volume is 3 litres.

Urinalysis   Ketones +

His 9-am investigations are as follows:

Hb	15 g/dL
WCC	11 × 10⁹/L
Platelets	469 × 10⁹/L
Sodium	140 mmol/L
Potassium	3.6 mmol/L
Bicarbonate	28 mmol/L
Chloride	100 mmol/L
Urea	7.0 mmol/L
Creatinine	112 µmol/L
Albumin	46 g/L
Glucose	4.2 mmol/L
Cortisol	300 nmol/L
Free T$_4$	13.3 pmol/L
TSH	1.2 mU/L
Plasma osmolality	294 mosmol/kg
Urine osmolality	303 mosmol/kg

Time	Urine volume in previous hour (mL)	Urine osmolality (mosmol/kg)	Weight (kg)	Plasma osmolality (mosmol/kg)
07.30			83	
08.00				284
08.30	150	200	82.9	
11.00				287
11.30	145	247	82.4	
13.30		296	82.0	
14.00				292
14.30	140	386	81.5	
15.30	145	405	81.2	296
2 µg DDAVP given intramuscularly				
16.30	100	570	81.4	295
17.30	70	912	82.2	288
18.30	40	987	82.8	286
19.30	50	932	82.8	286

1   What is the diagnosis?

- [ ] A   Nephrogenic diabetes insipidus
- [ ] B   Polyuric renal failure
- [x] C   Cranial diabetes insipidus   ✓
- [ ] D   Primary polydipsia
- [ ] E   None of the above

Case 4

A 60-year-old lady is seen in the clinic for hypercalcaemia. Shortly after the death of her husband 2 years ago, while being treated for depression, hypertension was noted; during the investigation of this a corrected calcium of 2.9 mmol/L was found, which has persisted. She has been well, apart from a Colles' fracture 9 years ago sustained when she slipped while ice-skating with her husband in Manhattan; she does not smoke or drink, eats a good diet and lives alone with her two greyhounds, one of which recently had a litter of puppies. She was adopted, did not know her parents and has no children.

On examination she is 167-cm tall, weighs 60 kg, has a blood pressure of 190/90 mmHg, with no postural drop, and no corneal calcification. Urinalysis is normal.

Her investigations are:

FBC	Normal
ESR	14 mm/h
Sodium	145 mmol/L
Potassium	4.4 mmol/L
Bicarbonate	18 mmol/L
Chloride	117 mmol/L
Urea	5.4 mmol/L
Creatinine	55 µmol/L
Calcium	3.02 mmol/L
Phosphate	0.7 mmol/L
ALP	100 U/L
Total protein	80 g/L
Globulins	39 g/L
Serum ACE	34 U/L
IgG	9.3 g/L
IgA	2.1 g/L
IgM	1.2 g/L
Electrophoresis	Normal
Plasma PTH	4.2 pmol/L

24-hour urine:

Volume	3900 mL
Creatinine	2.64 µmol/L
Calcium	2.35 mmol/L

1   What is the diagnosis?

- A   Raised anion gap metabolic acidosis
- B   Secondary hyperparathyroidism
- C   Multiple endocrine neoplasia (MEN) type 2A
- D   Familial hypercalcaemic hypocalciuria
- E   Primary hyperparathyroidism

Case 5

You are called to see a 68-year-old retired nurse who collapsed while having a lipoma removed from his back under a general anaesthetic. In the past he had Osgood Schlatter's disease. He is on no medication. His mother has type 1 diabetes, his two sisters are well.

On examination he is 1.88 m, weighs 80 kg, the pulse is 70 bpm, JVP 4 cm and blood pressure 110/70 mmHg with no postural drop. His capillary glucose was 1.8 mmol/L during the collapse but he came round within 10 minutes after having 25 g intravenous glucose.

The patient is shown in the following figure:

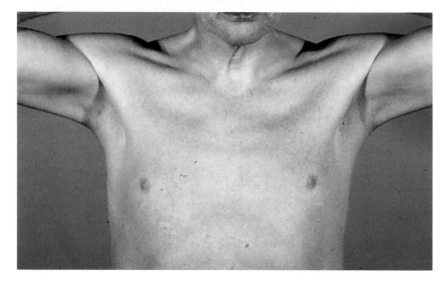

Urinalysis   Ketones ++

Prudently, some bloods were taken before the glucose was given. They are as follows:

FBC	Normal
Glucose	1.9 mmol/L
Sodium	135 mmol/L
Potassium	4.9 mmol/L
Bicarbonate	20 mmol/L
Chloride	104 mmol/L
Urea	3.5 mmol/L
Creatinine	70 µmol/L
LFTs	Normal
Cortisol	315 nmol/L

1   What is the next best step?

- [ ] A   Fast for up to 72 hours and measure insulin, C-peptide and β-hydroxybutyrate – if hypoglycaemia occurs
- [ ] B   Perform basal anterior pituitary function tests
- [ ] C   Urine or plasma sulphonylurea screen
- [ ] D   Short tetracosactrin test (250 μg Synacthen® intramuscularly, serum cortisol at 0, 30, 60 minutes)
- [ ] E   Measure plasma ACTH

Case 6

You see a 36-year-old lady 18 hours after her admission after palpitations which self-terminated. She is a gardener for the Royal Horticultural Society, smokes one or two cigarettes a week and drinks one bottle of wine every 2 days. She has no past medical history. She suffers with aches and pains all over which predate this presentation.

On examination the muscles are not tender and apart from being proximally weak – she cannot rise from a squat – the neurological examination, including the deep tendon reflexes, is normal; examination of the respiratory and abdominal systems are normal. The JVP is 4 cm and shows couplets of cannon waves and the BP is 140/94 mmHg.

Urinalysis	pH 6.1
	Protein trace
	Blood trace
	Specific gravity 1.010

The ECG shows U waves, but is otherwise entirely normal.

Her investigations are shown:

FBC	Normal
ESR	5 mm/h
CRP	<1 mg/L
Sodium	144 mmol/L
Potassium	2.2 mmol/L
Bicarbonate	6 mmol/L
Chloride	125 mmol/L
Urea	7.8 mmol/L
Creatinine	100 μmol/L
Calcium	2.2 mmol/L
Phosphate	0.7 mmol/L
Albumin	40 g/L
ALP	129 U/L
AST	22 U/L
ALT	15 U/L
Bilirubin	9 μmol/L

The ward house officer was concerned about some abdominal pain and requested the abdominal film shown opposite:

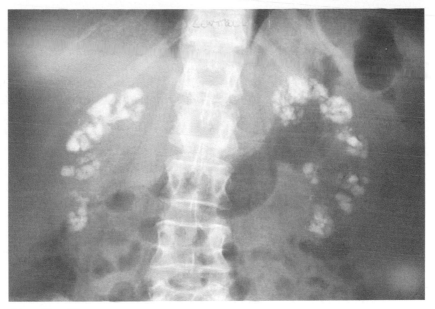

Science Photo Library

1   What is the diagnosis?

- [ ] A   Cushing's syndrome
- [ ] B   Distal renal tubular acidosis (type 1)
- [ ] C   Proximal renal tubular acidosis (type 2)
- [ ] D   Distal renal tubular acidosis (type 4)
- [ ] E   Primary aldosteronism (Conn's syndrome)

Case 7

A 29-year-old lady is admitted with a thunderclap frontal headache with severe pain behind the eyes. On direct questioning she had had some mild headaches for the preceding few days but had put that down to becoming increasingly exhausted over the previous months because of her work. She had double vision on looking to the left when the headache first came on. Recently she has lost 4 kg in weight. She takes no medications except the combined contraceptive pill.

On examination the temperature is 37.9 °C, pulse 110 bpm, BP 90/60 mmHg. She became too unsteady to get a standing BP. On examination of the external ocular movements she has a left VIth nerve palsy, but there are no other localising signs in the neurological examination. The discs are normal. Examination shows the breasts are normal and there is nothing to suggest a gynaecological malignancy.

She has a CT scan which does not show any blood and after 12 hours has a lumbar puncture:

Opening pressure	13 cmH$_2$O
CSF appearance	Clear and colourless
CSF microscopy:	
Lymphocytes	< 4/mm^3
Polymorphs	0
Red cells	0
CSF glucose	3.0 mmol/L
CSF protein	500 mg/L

Serum investigations are performed: ~~ADH !.~~

Sodium	120 mmol/L
Potassium	3.4 mmol/L
Urea	4 mmol/L
Creatinine	80 μmol/L
Serum osmolality	253 mosmol/kg
Urine osmolality	360 mosmol/kg

1   Which investigation will be most helpful?

- [ ] A   CT brain with contrast
- [ ] B   Cortisol and ACTH
- [ ] C   MRI pituitary
- [ ] D   Urinary sodium
- [x] E   CT orbit
- [ ] F   Send CSF to virology for examination before commencing aciclovir

Case 8

A 14-year-old boy is being investigated for the possibility of diabetes. He is fairly well and has not lost any weight. He had been treated for seborrhoeic eczema in the past without much success – the rash is still present. As a child, while in another country, he had been investigated for a soft-tissue mass on his head; the mass is still present. His mother has kept his X-rays from when he was a younger child and the skull X-ray is shown.

Urinalysis   Ketones +
                Specific gravity 1.002

His morning chemistry is shown:

Sodium	144 mmol/L	Plasma glucose	5.0 mmol/L
Potassium	4.0 mmol/L	Albumin	40 g/L
Chloride	108 mmol/L	ALP	300 U/L
Bicarbonate	26 mmol/L	ALT	30 U/L
Urea	3.0 mmol/L	Bilirubin	9 µmol/L
Creatinine	80 µmol/L		

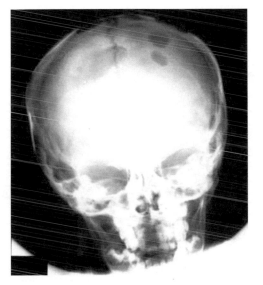

1   **What is the underlying diagnosis?**

☐   A   Primary hyperparathyroidism
☐   B   Multiple myeloma
☐   C   Langerhans' cell histiocytosis   ✗
☑   D   Neurofibromatosis type 1
☐   E   Metastatic carcinoma

Case 9

A 39-year-old lady attended for removal of a breast lump. Surgery was postponed because her BP was 200/110 mmHg, with no postural drop. She is on no medication and eats a normal diet. The JVP was 4 cm.

Urinalysis:

pH 7	
Ketones	Negative
Protein	Trace
Blood	Non-haemolysed trace

Your investigations reveal:

Sodium	140 mmol/L
Potassium	3.7 mmol/L
Bicarbonate	34 mmol/L
Chloride	96 mmol/L
Urea	6 mmol/L
Creatinine	110 µmol/L
Plasma renin activity	< 0.5 pmol/mL/h
Aldosterone	925 pmol/L

Urine:

Noradrenaline	500 nmol/24 h (NR < 570 nmol/24 h)
Adrenaline	90 nmol/24 h (NR < 144 nmol/24 h)
Dopamine	2000 nmol/24 h (3100 nmol/24 h)
Aldosterone	100 nmol/24 h

Ratio of cortisol/cortisone metabolites	Normal
Deoxycorticosterone (DOC)	Normal
β-HCG	Negative
Renal ultrasound	Normal

The adrenal CT is shown opposite.

1   What is the diagnosis?

☐   A   Primary aldosteronism – bilateral adrenal hyperplasia
☐   B   Liddle's syndrome
☐   C   Essential hypertension
☐   D   Bartter's syndrome
☐   E   Primary aldosteronism – unilateral adenoma
☐   F   Phaeochromocytoma

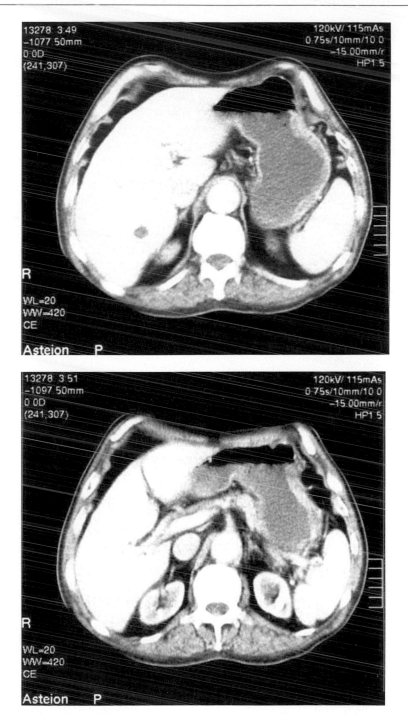

Case 10

A 49-year-old man with type 1 diabetes who is awaiting panretinal photocoagulation for proliferative retinopathy has central crushing chest pain with associated nausea and breathlessness. He has diabetic nephropathy, is on twice-daily Novomix-30®, with a recent HbA$_{1c}$ of 11.6% and had recently been advised to discontinue driving because of loss of hypoglycaemia awareness. His other medication is aspirin 75 mg once daily and 20 mg of simvastatin at night.

On examination he has a regular pulse of 88 bpm, the venous pressure is 4 cm, BP 95/68 mmHg, a third heart sound is present at the apex and the chest is clear. His ECG shows anterior ST elevation, suggestive of myocardial infarction. Primary angioplasty is unavailable.

The capillary glucose is 12.0 mmol/L

Urinalysis   Protein++

Investigations from the Diabetes Clinic the previous day show:

Sodium	135 mmol/L
Potassium	5.0 mmol/L
Bicarbonate	19 mmol/L
Urea	10.1 mmol/L
Creatinine	230 µmol/L
Glucose	12.6 mmol/L
Cholesterol	3.9 mmol/L
Bilirubin	10 µmol/L
Albumin	40 g/L
AST	105 U/L
ALT	100 U/L

1   Which of the following statements is incorrect?

- [ ] A Thrombolysis should be administered
- [ ] B β-Blockade should be given post-infarct
- [ ] C ACE inhibition should be given post-infarct
- [ ] D Intravenous β-blockade should not be given alongside thrombolysis
- [ ] E The statin should be discontinued

Case 11

A 39-year-old researcher at the European Parliament has abdominal and back pain which has come and gone for the last 18 months and is worsening. He smokes 20 cigarettes a day. He had always enjoyed wine while studying politics at university. However, because of the recurrent abdominal pain, he has not drunk for the last year. He has lost a little weight. He is not married.

On examination he weighs 68 kg and is 1.88 m tall. There is no spinal tenderness. The capillary glucose is 7.9 mmol/L.

Urinalysis	pH 6
Specific gravity	1.020

Investigations reveal:

Hb	12.1 g/dL
WCC	5.0×10^9/L
MCV	97 fL
Platelets	150×10^9/L
Bilirubin	42 μmol/L
Albumin	36 g/L
ALP	200 U/L
ALT	20 U/L
Amylase	100 U/L
Vitamin D	35 nmol/L (NR 45–90 nmol/l)
Cortisol	200 nmol/L

His spinal X-ray is shown overleaf.

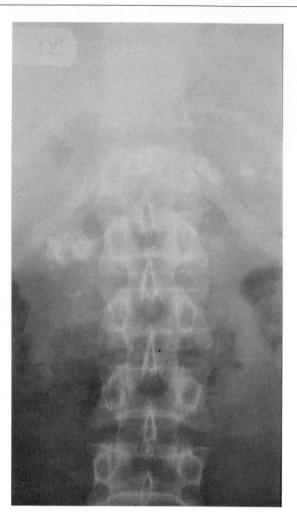

1   What is the diagnosis?

☐ A   Bone metastases
☐ B   Osteomalacia
☐ C   Chronic pancreatitis
☐ D   Carcinoma of the head of the pancreas
☐ E   Tuberculous adrenalitis

Case 12

You see a 22-year-old man for a second opinion regarding his endocrinology investigations for lassitude, weakness and cramps after exercise. His serum cortisol had been measured at 170 nmol/L. He was always tired as a child and performed poorly at sports in part, his parents used to say to his annoyance, because he was always a frail, sickly child. He suffers with such severe cramp when climbing even a few stairs that he now always takes the lift. He does not smoke or drink.

On examination he is thin, 1.8 m tall and weighs 57 kg. The skin is normal, there is no goitre or lymphadenopathy. He has a pulse of 88 bpm and BP of 130/70 mmHg with no drop, and a normal respiratory and abdominal examination. His thighs are wasted, there is no fasciculation, he cannot rise from a squat, the reflexes and sensation are normal.

Urinalysis	Ketones +
	Protein negative
	Blood ++
	Specific gravity 1.021
	Glucose negative
	Bilirubin negative

Fasting 9-am investigations after exertion show:

Cortisol	600 nmol/L
ACTH	15 pmol/L (NR at 9 am < 18 pmol/L)
FBC	Normal
ESR	< 1 mm/h
Creatine kinase	300 U/L
Glucose	5.0 mmol/L
Bicarbonate	24 mmol/L
Urea	2.2 mmol/L
Creatinine	50 µmol/L
LDH	320 U/L
LFTs	Normal
Bone profile	Normal
Corrected Ca^{2+}	2.4 mmol/L
Urine microscopy	No red cells or casts seen
	Sparse granular and hyaline casts

1   What is the diagnosis?

☐ A Cushing's disease
☐ B Pompé's disease
☐ C Cyclical Cushing's syndrome
☐ D McArdle's disease
☐ E Addison's disease

Case 13

A 55-year-old man who is asymptomatic has on two separate occasions shown the following venous plasma biochemistry:

Random glucose   6.1 mmol/L
75-g glucose tolerance test:
T + 0   6.0 mmol/L
T + 120   2 hrs   11.0 mmol/L

1   What is the diagnosis?

- ☐ A Diabetes mellitus
- ☐ B Impaired fasting glucose   ✓
- ☑ C Impaired glucose tolerance
- ☐ D Normal
- ☑ E Impaired fasting glucose and impaired glucose tolerance

Case 14

You are asked to see a 70-year-old lady on the Orthopaedic Ward who fractured her hip. She is 24 hours post-op from a dynamic hip screw insertion under general anaesthesia and is mildly nauseated but able to keep water down. She has COPD, well controlled on inhalers, and takes aspirin and a nitrate for mild stable angina – which has not troubled her for 'years'.

On examination she is orientated, pale, apyrexial, pulse 96 bpm, BP 90/50 mmHg lying and 96 bpm and 90/50 mmHg standing, and the JVP is 3 cm. Her chest is clear.

Urinalysis
Blood negative
Protein negative
Ketones +
pH 5.4

Her morning investigations are as follows:

Hb	9.9 g/dL
MCV	90 fL
Platelets	604×10^9/L
Sodium	124 mmol/L
Potassium	5.1 mmol/L
Bicarbonate	22 mmol/L
Chloride	100 mmol/L
Urea	3.1 mmol/L
Creatinine	50 µmol/L
Calcium	2.4 mmol/L
Phosphate	1.1 mmol/L
Albumin	40 g/L
T_4	15.1 pmol/L
TSH	2.1 U/L
Cortisol	120 nmol/L
Glucose	4.3 mmol/L
Urine osmolality	180 mosmol/kg
Plasma osmolality	271 mosmol/kg

1   Which of these is the best treatment?

- [ ] A   Restrict fluids to 500 mL/day
- [ ] B   Intravenous 0.9% saline 80–125 mL/h
- [ ] C   Hydrocortisone 100 mg intramuscularly 6-hourly and fludrocortisone 50–100 µg orally bd
- [ ] D   Hydrocortisone 100 mg intravenously stat and 20 mg orally tds
- [ ] E   DDAVP 1 µg intramuscularly stat

Case 15

A 32-year-old man had a rather sudden onset of sore throat, dysphagia and pain in the right ear 2 weeks previously. He is anxious, tremulous and sweaty.

On examination he has a fine tremor, the palms are moist and warm, the temperature is 38 °C, pulse 112 bpm and collapsing, BP 120/70 mmHg, and JVP 4 cm. In the neck there is a tender, slightly irregular, firm goitre with the right lobe being the larger; the overlying skin is faintly erythematous.

This is the appearance of his eyes:

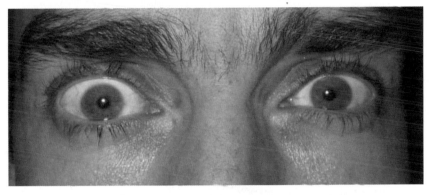

Investigations reveal:

Hb	12.0 g/dL
WCC	12.0 × 10⁹/L ↑
Platelets	397 × 10⁶/L
ESR	68 mm/h ↑

1   What is the likely diagnosis?

- ☐ A   Haemorrhage into a cyst
- ☐ B   Iodine-induced thyrotoxicosis (Jod–Basedow phenomenon)
- ☑ C   Subacute thyroiditis
- ☐ D   Graves' disease
- ☐ E   Riedel's thyroiditis

2   What is the diagnostic investigation?

- ☐ A   Free T₄, free T₃ and TSH
- ☐ B   Thyroglobulin
- ☑ C   Ultrasound and fine-needle aspiration (FNA)
- ☑ D   Radioactive iodine uptake scan
- ☐ E   Thyroid autoantibodies

Case 16

You are asked to see a 44-year-old Irish lady who is under investigation for colicky abdominal pain, nausea and vomiting, and lassitude which all come and go somewhat. She is a university lecturer who has been unwell with these symptoms over the last 9 months but has continued to work; she has lost 10 kg.

On examination she is 1.70 m tall and 57 kg and looks unwell. The pulse is 90 bpm, BP 120/80 mmHg lying and 90/52 mmHg standing, JVP 2 cm. Examination of the breasts, respiratory, abdominal and neurological systems is normal.

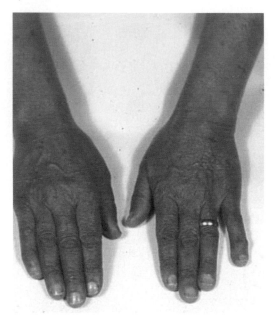

Her CXR is normal.

Morning investigations are performed:

Sodium	130 mmol/L
Potassium	6.3 mmol/L
Urea	10 mmol/L
Creatinine	110 μmol/L
Cortisol	210 nmol/L
ACTH	190 pmol/L (NR at 9 am < 18 pmol/L)
T_4	15.1 pmol/L
TSH	3.1 mU/L

1   Which test should be performed next?

- A   Short tetracosactrin (Synacthen®) test – 250 µg tetracosactrin intramuscularly at time 0
- B   Long tetracosactrin test – 1 mg tetracosactrin deep intramuscular injection at time 0
- C   Very-long-chain fatty acids
- D   Adrenal cortex and 21-hydroxylase autoantibodies
- E   Insulin tolerance test – 0.15 U/kg insulin at time 0

Case 17

A 32-year-old lady is seen in the Diabetes Clinic for 6-monthly review. She has had type 1 diabetes mellitus (T1DM) for the last 15 years. She is treated with insulin aspart 8–12 units pre-meal and human Insulatard® 18 units at 10 pm. She monitors frequently and while some days can be good with fasting capillary glucose in the range of 4.5–6.5 mmol/L and post-prandial levels of no higher than 9.5 mmol/L, she can wake with fasting sugars around 12–15 mmol/L and then the whole day is erratic. She always has a bedtime snack and she suspects she is having nocturnal hypoglycaemia. The HbA$_{1c}$ is 7.2% and she has no demonstrable complications. She is having no meter or pen problems.

On examination her weight is stable at 70 kg and she has a BMI of 22 kg/m^2; the injection sites are fine.

Investigations reveal:

Tissue transglutamase antibodies	Negative
9-am cortisol	400 nmol/L
β-HCG	< 5 U/L

1 What do you recommend?

- [ ] A Decrease the dose of the evening pre-meal aspart
- [ ] B Decrease the dose of the nocturnal Insulatard®
- [ ] C Add metformin
- [ ] D Change the nocturnal Insulatard® to insulin glargine
- [ ] E Perform a short tetracosactrin test

Case 18

A gentleman has been investigated for hip/thigh pain. This is his pelvic X-ray:

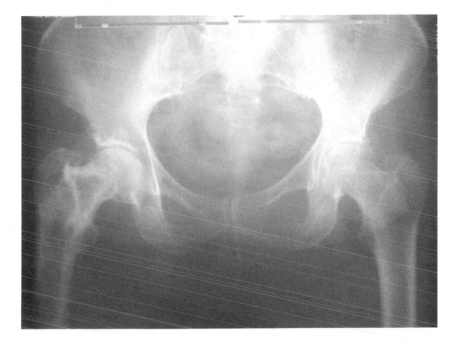

1   What is the likely diagnosis?

- A   Hyperparathyroidism
- B   Osteomalacia
- C   Acromegaly
- D   Metastatic prostate carcinoma
- E   Paget's disease

Case 19

This gentleman's foot is warm, swollen and red, but is not painful.

On examination the skin is intact – there is no ulceration. The foot is not tender. Peripheral pulses are present.

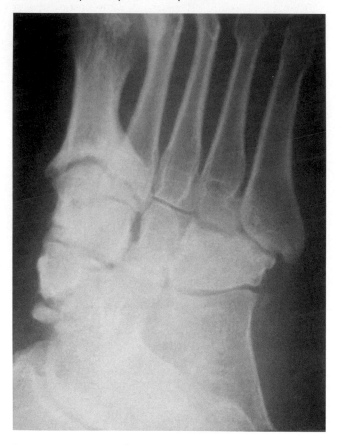

Investigations reveal:

Plasma glucose   15 mmol/L
Urate   400 mmol/L

1   What is the likely diagnosis?

- [ ] A   Acromegaly
- [ ] B   Gout
- [ ] C   Charcot's foot
- [ ] D   Osteomyelitis
- [ ] E   Cushing's syndrome

2 **What is the appropriate next step?**

- ☐ A Intravenous amoxicillin and flucloxacillin
- ☐ B Colchicine ± subsequent allopurinol
- ☐ C Growth hormone day-curve and check insulin-like growth factor-I (IGF-I) levels
- ☐ D Low-dose (0.5 mg 6-hourly for 48 hours) dexamethasone suppression test
- ☑ E Immobilisation and forbid weight-bearing

Case 20

This 45-year-old lady is seen in the Diabetes Clinic. She is currently only taking metformin 1 g bd, rosiglitazone 4 mg once daily and amlodipine 10 mg once daily. She does not smoke.

On examination her BMI is 32 kg/m² and she has a blood pressure of 150/90 mmHg. Examination of the praecordium, respiratory and abdominal systems is normal.

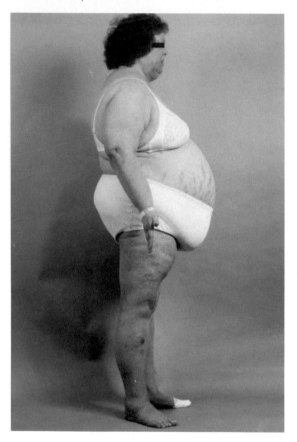

| Urinalysis | Glucose negative |
| | Blood ++ (menstruating) |

Fasting investigations:

HbA$_{1c}$	8.0%
Plasma glucose	5.9 mmol/L
Cholesterol	4.1 mmol/L
LDL cholesterol	3.0 mmol/L
HDL cholesterol	0.7 mmol/L
Triglycerides	2.1 mmol/L
Bilirubin	12 μmol/L
Albumin	37 g/L
ALT	60 U/L
AST	50 U/L
ALP	121 U/L
γGT	50 U/L
Prothrombin time	15.1 s
HBsAg	Negative
Hepatitis C virus Ab	Negative

Ultrasound of the liver shows no biliary dilatation.

1   What is the likely diagnosis?

- [x] A   Cushing's syndrome
- [ ] B   Normal glucose tolerance
- [ ] C   Adrenal carcinoma
- [ ] D   Haemochromatosis
- [ ] E   Rosiglitazone-induced hepatitis

2   Which two are the appropriate next steps?

- [ ] A   Stop the rosiglitazone
- [ ] B   Increase the rosiglitazone
- [ ] C   Stop the metformin and the rosiglitazone
- [ ] D   Endoscopic retrograde cholangiopancreatography (ERCP)
- [x] E   MRI pituitary
- [ ] F   Serum ferritin
- [x] G   Midnight serum cortisol
- [x] H   Prescribe a statin
- [ ] I   Liver biopsy
- [ ] J   48-hour low-dose dexamethasone suppression test

Case 21

This 50-year-old gentleman has macular degeneration, the opthalmologist asks you to see him as his blood pressure is 150/100 mmHg. This is his right hand:

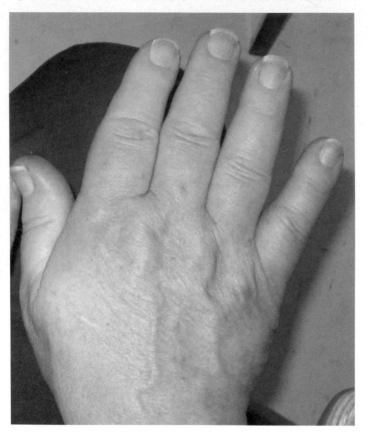

1   Which two diagnostic tests will you perform on him?

☐   A   Growth hormone day curve
☐   B   X-ray hands
☐   C   Anti-nuclear and extractable nuclear antibodies
☑   D   Measure growth hormone during an oral glucose tolerance test
☑   E   Pituitary MRI
☐   F   Measure growth hormone during an insulin tolerance test
☐   G   Serum alkaline phosphatase
☐   H   Serum urate
☐   I   Rheumatoid factor
☐   J   Serum albumin

Case 22

This 49-year-old lady complains of nocturia for the past 6 months:

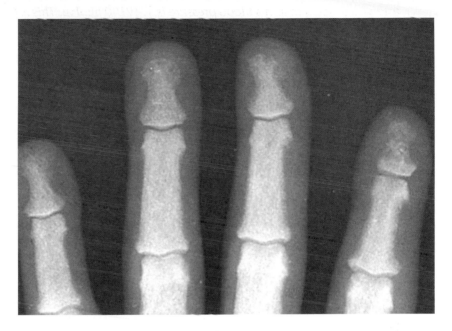

1   What is the diagnosis?

- [ ] A   Acromegaly
- [ ] B   Diabetic cheiroarthropathy
- [ ] C   Osteoarthritis
- [ ] D   Hyperparathyroidism
- [ ] E   Osteomalacia

Case 23

A GP refers you a 65-year-old gentleman with breathlessness which has been present and slowly worsening for the last few weeks. The GP is concerned that there is something he is missing. The patient is not wheezy but has had a cough productive of green sputum for the last 2 days that has not responded to amoxicillin as well as normally; the GP had treated him for several infections, including pneumonia twice and urinary tract infections over the preceding months. He normally has a cough productive of white sputum. He has lost 5 kg in weight over the last 3 months and on direct questioning says he lost his appetite, is not sleeping and is feeling frankly miserable. There have been no night sweats. No prescription medication is taken but he takes magnesium trisilicate several times daily for a very troublesome hiatus hernia; he is married with two grown-up children, recently retired as a bank clerk, drinks approximately 30 units of alcohol a week and keeps no pets.

On examination he is thin, pale and looks a little unwell. His respiratory rate is 24 breaths per minute, the chest is clear and there is no wheeze. The pulse is 96 bpm, BP 130/70 mmHg and the heart, abdomen and nervous system are normal.

Urinalysis	Protein negative
Sputum	Thick, green, purulent
SpO_2	94%

Investigations:

Hb	8.8 g/dL
MCV	84 fL
WCC	3.1×10^9/L
Neutrophils	1.1×10^9/L
Lymphocytes	2.0×10^9/L
Platelets	120×10^9/L
ESR	110 mm/h
Sodium	139 mmol/L
Potassium	4.9 mmol/L
Bicarbonate	19 mmol/L
Chloride	106 mmol/L
Urea	19.1 mmol/L
Creatinine	180 μmol/L
Calcium	2.7 mmol/L
Phosphate	1.8 mmol/L
Albumin	26 g/L
ALP	90 U/L
Total protein	78 g/L

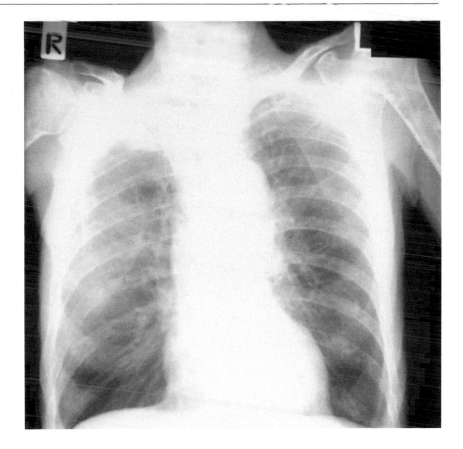

1   What is the diagnosis?

- [ ] A Squamous cell carcinoma of the lung
- [ ] B Multiple myeloma
- [ ] C Bone metastases
- [ ] D Hyperparathyroidism
- [ ] E Milk alkali syndrome

Case 24

A local GP has asked you to see a 29-year-old lady who complains of palpitations which have been present for the last 2 months. She has diarrhoea.

The GP had her thyroid function tests assayed at a local district general hospital 3 months ago which revealed:

Free T$_4$ 30.1 pmol/L
Free T$_3$ 12.9 pmol/L
TSH   4.3 mU/L

When you see her the pulse is 110 bpm and she has a small goitre. Urine β-HCG is negative.

On the assay at your hospital the investigations reveal:

Free T$_4$ 32.1 pmol/L
Free T$_3$ 14.1 pmol/L
TSH   4.9 mU/L

1   What is the appropriate next step?

☐   A   Serum β-HCG
☐   B   Repeat the tests
☐   C   Pituitary MRI
☐   D   Thyrotrophin-releasing hormone (TRH) test
☐   E   Check serum cortisol

Case 25

A 52-year-old journalist, who has been followed up in the Diabetes Clinic since diagnosis 3 years ago, is brought to A&E with a gastrointestinal bleed. His diabetes is always fairly well controlled on metformin 850 mg bd and pioglitazone 15 mg once daily with an HbA$_{1c}$ of 6.9%. He does not smoke but likes to have a couple of whiskeys while listening to the radio in the evening. He is married with three children who are well. His father had diabetes mellitus and died of heart failure at 49 years of age. He is otherwise well, apart from some arthritis in his knees, for which he takes simple analgesia.

On examination he has pale conjunctivae, is tanned and has abdominal obesity and swollen knees. His pulse is 120 bpm and chaotic, BP 110/90 mmHg with postural symptoms. There is 3-cm hepatomegaly. The chest is normal and he has absent ankle jerks. You resuscitate him appropriately.

Investigations:

Hb	9.0 g/dL
WCC	10 × 10^9/L
MCV	90 fL
Platelets	90 × 10^9/L
Prothrombin time	19 s
Fibrinogen	1.8 g/L
Albumin	32 g/L
ALT	90 U/L
AST	90 U/L
γGT	120 U/L
Bilirubin	23 μmol/L
Creatine kinase	140 U/L

He has an endoscopy in the morning, showing varices which are banded.

1   What is the diagnosis?

- [ ] A   Simvastatin-induced hepatitis
- [ ] B   Haemochromatosis
- [ ] C   Rosiglitazone-induced liver failure
- [ ] D   Alcoholic cirrhosis
- [ ] E   NSAID-induced peptic ulceration

Case 26

A patient presents showing the following changes on X-ray:

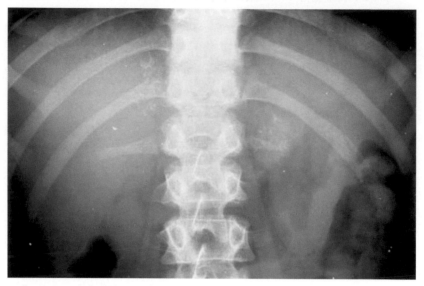

Wellcome Trust Medical Photographic Library

1   What biochemical abnormalities would you expect in this patient?

☐   A   Elevated renin, normal anion gap acidosis, hyperkalaemia, high TSH
☐   B   Hypercalcaemia, normal anion gap acidosis, hypophosphataemia
☐   C   Elevated renin, high aldosterone, hypokalaemia, alkalosis
☐   D   Low potassium, low chloride, hypophosphataemia, elevated alkaline
           phosphatase
☐   E   Hypokalaemia, elevated plasma catecholamines, hyperglycaemia

Case 27

You suspect that a 55-year-old lady with hypertension, dyslipidaemia, diabetes mellitus and osteoporosis has Cushing's syndrome based on suspicious appearance; you perform some investigations:

9 am cortisol	590 nmol/L
Cortisol after 48 hours of dexamethasone 0.5 mg 6-hourly	290 nmol/L
Cortisol after 48 hours of dexamethasone 2 mg 6-hourly	140 nmol/L
Plasma ACTH awaited	

1   What is the likely diagnosis?

- ☐ A Ectopic ACTH secretion
- ☐ B Adrenal carcinoma
- ☑ C Cushing's disease ✓
- ☐ D Adrenal adenoma
- ☐ E Normal

Case 28

A 24-year-old patient is seen in the clinic with type 1 diabetes of 11 years' duration. His glycaemia is acceptable on insulin detemir 10 units bd and insulin aspart 8, 10, 8 pre-meal – the HbA$_{1c}$ is 7.4%. He has background retinopathy which is under follow-up and mild asymptomatic peripheral sensory neuropathy. He had an albumin/creatinine ratio (ACR) of 2.9 mg/mmol 6 weeks ago at his surgery. He does not smoke.

On examination his weight is 69.1 kg and BMI 20 kg/m². Blood pressure is 128/78 mmHg. He has microaneurysms, blot haemorrhages and four hard exudates in the periphery; the acuity is 6/6 bilaterally.

Urinalysis	Protein negative
	Blood negative

Investigations:

First morning urine albumin/creatinine ratio	2.7 mg/mmol
Total cholesterol	3.6 mmol/L
HDL cholesterol	1.3 mmol/L
LDL cholesterol	2.2 mmol/L
Triglycerides	1.8 mmol/L
Creatinine	80 µmol/L

1   What should you do?

- [ ] A   Start aspirin, a standard dose of statin and start an ACE inhibitor and titrate to the maximum dose
- [x] B   Start an ACE inhibitor and titrate to the maximum dose
- [ ] C   Start aspirin and an ACE and titrate to the maximum dose
- [ ] D   Start aspirin alone
- [ ] E   Start an ACE inhibitor, titrate to the maximum dose and refer to an ophthalmologist for laser photocoagulation

Case 29

A 69-year-old Asian gentleman is seen in Outpatients after a recent stent to his left anterior descending artery. He is pain-free. He takes atenolol 100 mg once daily, amlodipine 10 mg once daily, ramipril 10 mg once daily, aspirin 75 mg once daily, clopidogrel 75 mg once daily, metformin 850 mg tds, pioglitazone 15 mg and atorvastatin 80 mg at night. He had pancreatitis caused by hypertriglyceridaemia 3 years ago when his diabetes mellitus was diagnosed; he was taking colestyramine at that time. He is an ex-smoker and takes no alcohol.

On examination, BP is 120/70 mmHg and BMI 28 kg/m².

You are asking the dietician to see him again.

These are his lipids:

Total cholesterol	5.4 mmol/L
LDL cholesterol	3.2 mmol/L
HDL cholesterol	1.2 mmol/L
Triglycerides	1.9 mmol/L
Creatine kinase	100 U/L
ALT	25 U/L
AST	20 U/L
HbA_{1c}	6.9%

1   Which of the following is the most prudent?

- ☐ A   Add a fish oil
- ☐ B   Add a fibrate
- ☐ C   Re-challenge with colestyramine
- ☐ D   Add nicotinic acid
- ☐ E   Add ezetimibe

Case 30

A 72-year-old gentleman is admitted to hospital after collapsing in the street, outside his house. The initial diagnosis is a stroke as he has a dense right hemiparesis. His conscious level is decreased and details are initially scarce. His fingers are tar-stained. Your computer system tells you he is seen in the Movement Disorder Clinic and was admitted 5 months ago for 5 days under the geriatricians.

On examination he is responsive only to pain, and tolerating a Guedel's airway. He has generalised obesity and is pale. His is cool round the peripheries, the pulse is 60 bpm and chaotic, BP 120/90 mmHg, the apex is impalpable but the heart sounds are normal, the respiratory rate is 16 breaths per minute, there are coarse crackles posteriorly at the bases to the mid-zones with bronchial breathing, the abdomen is distended but there is no organomegaly. The ankle jerks are absent. SpO_2 is 94%. Capillary glucose is 4.1 mmol/L.

Initial investigations reveal:

Hb	13.1 g/dL
MCV	98 fL
WCC	10.1×10^9/L
Platelets	200×10^9/L
Sodium	122 mmol/L
Potassium	3.5 mmol/L
Urea	12.1 mmol/L
Creatinine	124 mmol/L
Serum osmolality	267 mosmol/kg

His chest X-rays are shown opposite.

Chest X-ray, 5 months ago

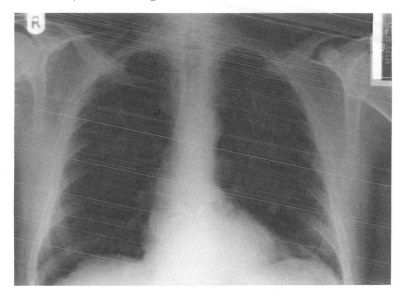

Chest X-ray, now

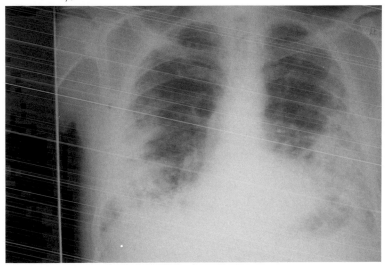

1   What is responsible for this appearance?

☐   A   Aspiration pneumonia
☐   B   Amiodarone
☐   C   Lithium
☐   D   Cabergoline
☐   E   Demeclocycline

Case 31

A 62-year-old man is admitted after a collapse. He has a 'turn' on the ward and his capillary glucose is found to be 2.2 mmol/L. With 50 mL of 50% dextrose he recovers rapidly and the capillary glucose rises to 7 mmol/L. He goes on to have a 72-hour fast.

Urinalysis	No abnormalities detected

These are the data after 18 hours of fasting, when he becomes unwell:

Glucose	2.1 mmol/L
Insulin	40 pmol/L
C peptide	500 pmol/L
Cortisol	580 nmol/L
Plasma sulphylureas	Absent
Growth hormone	44 mU/L (NR basal, fasting and between pulses < 1 mU/L, after hypoglycaemia > 40 mU/L)
Prolactin	300 mU/L (NR < 360 mU/L)
Calcium	2.4 mmol/L
Albumin	40 g/L

1   What is the correct cause?

- [ ] A   Exogenous insulin administration
- [ ] B   Non-islet-cell hypoglycaemia
- [ ] C   Insulinoma
- [ ] D   Multiple endocrine neoplasia type 1 (MEN 1)
- [ ] E   Sulphonylurea or nate/repa-glinide administration

Chapter Three

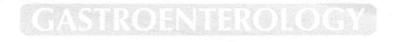

GASTROENTEROLOGY

Case 1

A 55-year-old man diagnosed with total ulcerative colitis at the age of 20 presented with a 3-month history of rectal bleeding. He was opening his bowels twice a day, passing formed stool. His colitis had been well-controlled for the last 10 years with oral mesalazine 400 mg bd.

His blood tests were as follows:

Hb	8.6 g/dL
MCV	75 fL
WCC	4.8×10^9/L
Platelets	387×10^9/L
CRP	5 mg/L

1   What is the most appropriate next step?

- ☐   A   Oral prednisolone 40 mg/day
- ☐   B   Increase oral mesalazine to 800 mg tds
- ☐   C   Colectomy
- ☐   D   Colonoscopy
- ☐   E   Azathioprine 2 mg/kg/day

Case 2

Four weeks after returning from a trip to the Indian subcontinent, a 44-year-old woman presented to A&E complaining that she had been feeling unwell for about a week with symptoms of nausea and anorexia. She did not drink alcohol, took no regular medications and had had only one sexual partner for the last few years. There was no past medical history of note.

Examination revealed a tender liver, palpable to 4 cm below the costal margin. The spleen was also just palpable. Blood results were as follows:

Sodium	139 mmol/L
Potassium	3.7 mmol/L
Urea	2.8 mmol/L
Creatinine	76 µmol/L
Albumin	35 g/L
Bilirubin	21 µmol/L
AST	345 U/L
ALT	755 U/L
ALP	256 U/L
Hepatitis A	IgG positive
Hepatitis A	IgM negative

1   Which of the following is the most likely diagnosis?

☐   A   Acute hepatitis A
☐   B   Acute hepatitis C
☐   C   Chronic hepatitis A
☐   D   Acute hepatitis B
☐   E   Acute hepatitis E

Case 3

A 24-year-old lady with an 8-year history of ileocolonic Crohn's disease presented with a 2-day history of shortness of breath. She had smoked 10 cigarettes a day for the last 10 years. Her Crohn's disease had been difficult to control and she had recently been started on oral prednisolone, 40 mg per day, in addition to her usual medications of oral mesalazine and methotrexate, both of which she had been taking for many years.

On examination she had a respiratory rate of 22 breaths/minute and her pulse was 110 bpm. Auscultation of her chest was unremarkable.

1   Which of the following tests is the most appropriate?

☐   A   Plain chest X-ray
☐   B   Ventilation–perfusion scan
☐   C   Pulmonary function tests
☐   D   D-dimer levels
☐   E   Lung biopsy

Case 4

A 31-year-old lady presents with a 2-month history of malaise and anorexia. She drinks 21 units of alcohol a week and returned from a holiday in South-East Asia 3 months previously. She is on no regular medication and has not had any recent sexual contacts.

Her investigations were as follows:

Hb	11.6 g/dL
MCV	87 fL
WCC	4.8×10^9/L
Platelets	115×10^9/L
Bilirubin	30 µmol/L
ALT	345 U/L
Albumin	36 g/L
ALP	124 U/L
Total protein	90 g/L

1   What is the most likely diagnosis?

☐   A   Autoimmune hepatitis
☐   B   Hepatitis A virus infection
☐   C   Alcoholic liver disease
☐   D   Gallstones
☐   E   Primary biliary cirrhosis

Case 5

A 64-year-old lady presented with a 2 day history of melaena and epigastric pain. She had a history of osteoarthritis for which she took diclofenac.

On admission she had a pulse of 125 bpm. Her blood pressure was 110/70 mmHg lying and 100/50 mmHg when sitting. She was resuscitated with intravenous colloid. At endoscopy, she was found to have a stricture in the mid-oesophagus which prevented passage of the endoscope. She continued to have melaena and accordingly had angiography performed which is shown below.

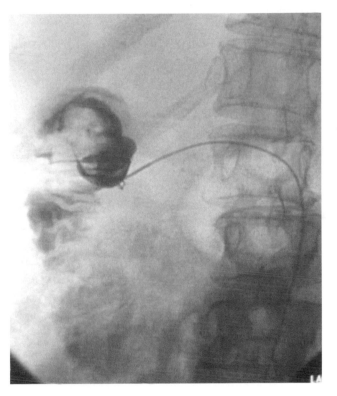

1   What is the most likely source of her bleeding?

- ☐ A   Oesophageal carcinoma
- ☐ B   Aortoenteric fistula
- ☐ C   Oesophageal varices
- ☐ D   Duodenal ulcer
- ☐ E   Meckel's diverticulum

Case 6

A 42-year-old man is referred to Outpatients with a history of tiredness. He had previously had a prophylactic colectomy with ileostomy formation for a family history of colorectal carcinoma.

The specimen from this operation is shown below. His ileostomy is functioning normally and external examination is unremarkable.

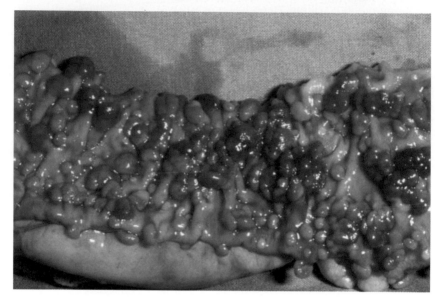

His blood tests are as follows:

Hb	8.6 g/dl
MCV	72 fL
WCC	4.8×10^9/L
Platelets	411×10^9/L

1   What is the most likely diagnosis?

☐ A   Vitamin B_{12} malabsorption secondary to his resection
☐ B   Malabsorption of iron secondary to his resection
☐ C   Duodenal carcinoma
☐ D   Abdominal desmoids
☐ E   Pernicious anaemia

Case 7

A 28-year-old woman of Irish descent was referred to hospital with a history of malaise and tiredness for 6 months. She complained that her bowels had always been erratic but were more so recently; she had been passing semi-formed stools three times a day for the last few months. There was no history of foreign travel and, other than the oral contraceptive pill, she was on no regular medications.

Examination revealed that she was pale and undernourished. Her laboratory investigations were as follows:

Hb	9.6 g/dL
MCV	74 fL
WCC	6.2×10^9/L
Platelets	221×10^9/L
Sodium	139 mmol/L
Potassium	3.7 mmol/L
Urea	2.8 mmol/L
Creatinine	76 µmol/L
Albumin	33 g/L
Calcium	1.76 mmol/L
Bilirubin	5 µmol/L
AST	23 U/L
ALP	94 U/L

Anti-endomysial Ab negative

1   What is the most appropriate test?

- [ ] A   Capsule endoscopy
- [ ] B   Barium follow through
- [ ] C   Duodenal aspiration for parasites
- [ ] D   Serum IgA levels
- [ ] E   Distal duodenal biopsy

Case 8

A 74-year-old woman presented with a 4-month history of anorexia and weight loss. She had previously been fit and well and, apart from some mild epigastric pain, had no other symptoms.

On examination she was clinically anaemic and had an area of abnormal pigmentation on the back (see below).

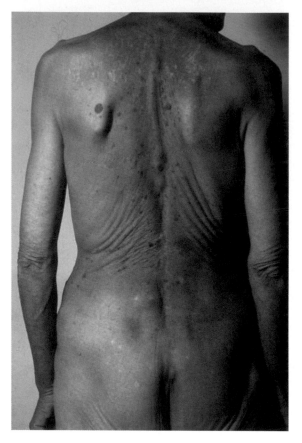

1   What is the most likely diagnosis?

- [ ] A   Duodenal ulceration
- [ ] B   Coeliac disease
- [ ] C   Dietary folate deficiency
- [ ] D   Crohn's disease
- [ ] E   Gastric carcinoma

Case 9

A 35-year-old woman was referred to hospital with a 6-month history of diarrhoea. She described the passage of watery stool up to five times a day with associated cramping lower abdominal pain and bloating. There was no history of foreign travel or of weight loss, and she did not take any regular medications.

Examination of the perianal region revealed some excoriation but digital rectal examination and rigid sigmoidoscopy were normal. Her investigations were as follows:

Hb	13.5 g/dL
MCV	90 fL
WCC	5.8×10^9/L
Platelets	387×10^9/L
Sodium	138 mmol/L
Potassium	4.2 mmol/L
Urea	2.4 mmol/L
Creatinine	99 µmol/L
Albumin	44 g/L
Corrected Ca^{2+}	2.4 mmol/L
Bilirubin	14 µmol/L
CRP	5 mg/L

1   What is the most likely diagnosis?

- ☐ A   Coeliac disease
- ☐ B   Crohn's disease
- ☐ C   Small-bowel bacterial overgrowth
- ☐ D   Infectious diarrhoea
- ☐ E   Bile-salt malabsorption

Case 10

A 42-year-old lady presented to A&E with a 4-week history of fevers, malaise, headache and a cough productive of yellow sputum. She had also noted occasional fevers and had lost 3 kg in weight. She had a 20-year history of small-bowel and perianal fistulating Crohn's disease for which she was taking azathioprine (2 mg/kg) and had recently had her second infusion of anti-tumour necrosis factor-α antibodies. Her diarrhoea and abdominal pain had improved and the perianal fistulae had become less active. She smoked 20 cigarettes a day and had done so for 15 years.

On examination, her temperature was 37.4 °C and her chest had occasional scattered wheezes throughout. Her abdomen was soft and non-tender. Her chest X-ray is shown below.

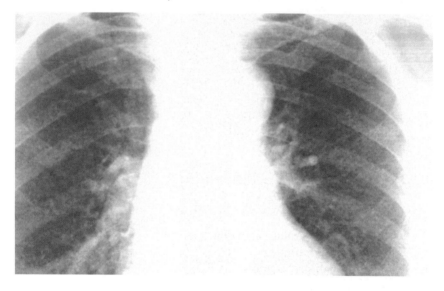

1   What is the likely diagnosis?

☐   A   Tuberculosis
☐   B   Granulomatous lung disease
☐   C   Reaction to infliximab
☐   D   Lung cancer
☐   E   Pneumonia

Case 11

A 55-year-old man was referred by his GP with recent onset of dysphagia. Although able to swallow most of the time, he found that food stuck if he did not chew it adequately. He had a long history of gastro-oesophageal reflux for which he took a proton pump inhibitor, but he had never had an upper gastrointestinal endoscopy. He was otherwise asymptomatic. He had smoked 15 cigarettes a day for the last 40 years and drank two measures of whisky each night before bed.

Examination of his abdomen was unremarkable and all his blood tests were normal. A barium swallow was performed:

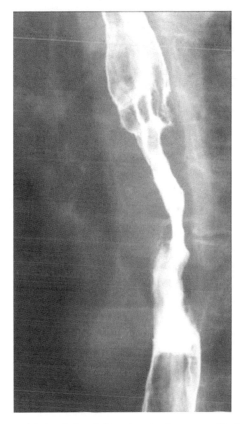

1   Which of the following is the most likely diagnosis?

- [ ] A   Diffuse oesophageal spasm
- [ ] B   Oesophageal carcinoma
- [ ] C   Achalasia
- [ ] D   Peptic stricturing
- [ ] E   Barrett's oesophagus

Case 12

A 44-year-old man was referred by his GP with a 2-month history of foul-smelling, greasy stools. He had recently returned from an 8-week trip to Vietnam, his symptoms having developed about halfway through his stay. His weight had decreased by 4 kg over the last 4 weeks. He was opening his bowels up to six times per day and had accompanying abdominal pain, bloating and nausea. He drank 28 units of alcohol per week and took multivitamins. External examination was unremarkable.

His GP had sent a stool sample for microscopy and culture, the results of which were normal.

1   **Which of the following organisms is most likely to account for his symptoms?**

☐ A   *Balantidium coli*
☐ B   *Entamoeba histolytica*
☐ C   *Giardia lamblia*
☐ D   *Cryptosporidium parvum*
☐ E   *Entamoeba coli*

Case 13

A 56-year-old Chinese woman presented to Outpatients with a history of nausea, upper abdominal pain, abdominal swelling and weight loss. There was no history of change in bowel habit or rectal bleeding and she had no past history of note.

Examination revealed jaundice, 4-cm, irregular hepatomegaly, and gross ascites. No other masses were palpable in her abdomen.

Serum tumour markers were as follows:

α-fetoprotein   200 ng/ml
CEA   2 μg/L
CA 125   900 U/mL

A CT scan of her abdomen is shown below.

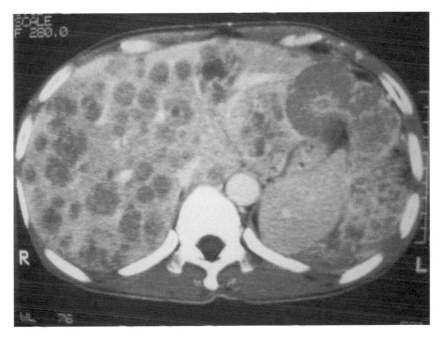

1   What is the most likely diagnosis?

- [ ] A Hydatid disease
- [ ] B Hepatocellular carcinoma
- [ ] C Metastatic ovarian cancer
- [ ] D Metastatic colonic cancer
- [ ] E Polycystic liver disease

Case 14

A 33-year-old lady presented to A&E with a 2-week history of nausea and vomiting, malaise and headache. She was 36 weeks pregnant and had had three uncomplicated pregnancies previously.

Examination revealed that she was normotensive and had mild peripheral oedema. Palpation of her abdomen revealed a gravid uterus consistent with the duration of her pregnancy and mild tenderness in her right upper quadrant. Her urine was negative for protein. Her blood tests were as follows:

Hb	8.6 g/dL
MCV	98 fL
WCC	5.8×10^9/L
Platelets	98×10^9/L
Sodium	138 mmol/L
Potassium	4.4 mmol/L
Urea	4.4 mmol/L
Creatinine	99 µmol/L
Albumin	32 g/L
Bilirubin	30 µmol/L
AST	1245 U/L
ALP	256 U/L

1   Which of the following is the most likely diagnosis?

- A   Acute fatty liver of pregnancy
- B   Hyperemesis gravidarum
- C   HELLP syndrome
- D   Intrahepatic cholestasis of pregnancy
- E   Pre-eclampsia

Case 15

A 52-year-old gentleman was admitted with a history of haematemesis. He had drunk ten cans of strong lager a day for the last 10 years.

Examination revealed that he was tachycardic (110 bpm) and hypotensive (95/60 mmHg supine). He was jaundiced and had multiple spider naevi on his chest wall. His spleen was palpable on inspiration and shifting dullness was detectable.

Blood results were as follows:

Hb	8.6 g/dL
MCV	104 fL
WCC	4.8×10^9/L
Platelets	77×10^9/L
PT	28 s
Sodium	129 mmol/L
Potassium	4.4 mmol/L
Urea	1.4 mmol/L
Creatinine	78 µmol/L
Albumin	23 g/l
Bilirubin	35 µmol/L
AST	245 U/l
ALP	256 U/L

1 **Which of the following is not appropriate as part of your immediate management?**

- A Upper gastrointestinal endoscopy
- B Propranolol
- C Intravenous Terlipressin
- D Intravenous antibiotics
- E Diagnostic peritoneal aspirate

Case 16

A 19-year-old Bangladeshi man was referred to Outpatients with a history of slight weight loss, crampy abdominal pain and, occasionally bloody diarrhoea. He smoked 20 cigarettes a day, drank 14 units of alcohol per week and worked as a mechanic. There was no past history of note. He had started taking ibuprofen for his abdominal pain and loperamide for his diarrhoea.

On examination he was well, apyrexial and not tachycardic. He had mild tenderness in his right iliac fossa but no masses were palpable in his abdomen. His barium follow-through is shown below.

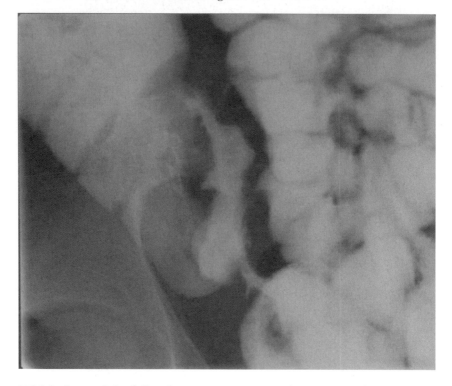

1   **Which three of the following are most appropriate as part of your initial management?**

☐ A Mesalazine
☐ B Stop smoking
☐ C Stop ibuprofen
☐ D Increase loperamide dosage
☐ E Azathioprine
☐ F Infliximab
☐ G Vitamin B_{12} injections
☐ H Methotrexate
☐ I Parenteral hydrocortisone
☐ J Surgery

Case 17

A 22-year-old student, who had recently returned from a holiday in South-East Asia, presents to A&E complaining of worsening abdominal pain following a 7-day history of bloody diarrhoea.

Examination revealed that he was pyrexial at 37.8 °C, sweaty and tachycardic at 105 bpm. His blood pressure was 95/55 mmHg and palpation of his abdomen revealed that he was diffusely tender. His plain abdominal X-ray is shown below.

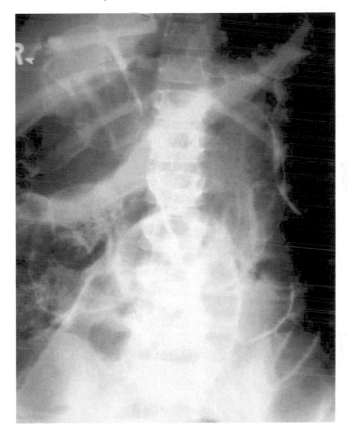

1   What should his subsequent management be?

- A   Referral to the surgical team for laparotomy
- B   Fluid resuscitation and antibiotics
- C   Fluid resuscitation and await stool cultures
- D   Sigmoidoscopy for deflation of the large bowel
- E   Fluid resuscitation, nil by mouth and nasogastric aspiration

Case 18

A 19-year-old woman was brought into hospital by her mother who had recently returned home to find that her daughter was unwell. Two days previously, the daughter had split up from her boyfriend and had taken about 50 paracetamol tablets after drinking a quarter of a bottle of spirits. She was not known to be a heavy drinker and had no past history of liver disease. Other than the oral contraceptive pill, she was on no regular medications.

On examination, her temperature was 37.1 °C. She was tearful and withdrawn, but alert and orientated. Aggressive fluid resuscitation and treatment with N-acetylcysteine were initiated.

1   **Which one of the following tests, taken the following day, should prompt referral to a specialist liver unit?**

☐   A   Paracetamol level 50 mg/L
☐   B   AST 856 U/L
☐   C   Albumin 22 g/L
☐   D   pH 7.25
☐   E   Creatinine 185 µmol/L

Case 19

A 65 year-old lady presented with a 6-month history of intermittent epigastric pain radiating to the back. For the past 2 weeks she had noticed that her stools had become pale and her urine dark. An ultrasound of her upper abdomen revealed that her common bile duct and intrahepatic ducts were dilated. She had had a cholecystectomy 15 years previously for cholelithiasis.

An image from endoscopic retrograde cholangiopancreatography (ERCP) is shown below.

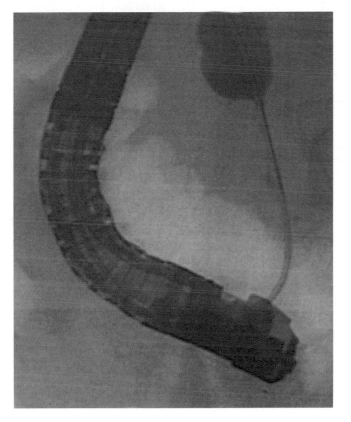

1   What is the most likely diagnosis?

- [ ] A   Ampullary carcinoma
- [ ] B   Retained stones in the biliary tree
- [ ] C   Pancreatic carcinoma
- [ ] D   Primary biliary cirrhosis
- [ ] E   Primary sclerosing cholangitis

Case 20

A 78-year-old woman was referred to Outpatients for an opinion. She lived in a nursing home and, along with many of the other residents, had had an attack of diarrhoea 10 weeks previously. However, her symptoms had persisted and she was still opening her bowels eight times a day and was now passing bloody stools. Over the last few days, lesions had been noted on her legs.

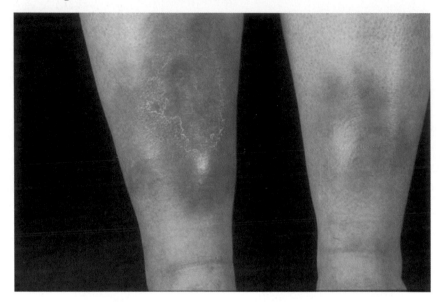

1   What is the lesion shown?

- ☐   A   Erythema nodosum
- ☐   B   Pyoderma gangrenosum
- ☐   C   Sweet's syndrome
- ☐   D   Dermatitis herpetiformis
- ☐   E   Acanthosis nigricans

2   What is the most likely diagnosis?

- ☐   A   Infective diarrhoea
- ☐   B   Carcinoma of the colon
- ☐   C   Coeliac disease
- ☐   D   Ulcerative colitis
- ☐   E   Ischaemic colitis

Case 21

A 31-year old lawyer was referred by his GP who had investigated him for tiredness. As part of a screen of blood tests he had been found to have abnormal liver function tests. He had occasionally used intravenous drugs as a student but had not done so recently. He was married and had had no other sexual partners for the last 4 years. Other than feeling tired, he was asymptomatic. He took no regular medications and drank 40 units of alcohol a week.

Blood tests were as follows:

Bilirubin	21 µmol/L
AST	85 U/L
ALT	165 U/L
ALP	112 U/L

Hepatitis serology:
Hepatitis A IgM negative
Hepatitis A IgG negative

HBsAg positive
HBeAg positive
Anti-HBc antibody positive
Anti HBe antibody negative

Hepatitis C virus antibody negative

1   Which one of the following is not part of the initial management?

- [ ] A   Vaccination against hepatitis A
- [ ] B   Hepatitis screening for his partner
- [ ] C   Liver biopsy
- [ ] D   Abstinence from alcohol
- [ ] E   Treatment with ribavirin

Case 22

A 78-year-old retired banker was reviewed in the Outpatients Department after a recent admission with right lower lobe pneumonia. She had had two similar episodes, managed by her GP, over the last 2 years. She had mild angina for which she was taking aspirin and atenolol. Otherwise she was fit and well. She smoked 15 cigarettes a day from the age of 20, and drank 15 units of alcohol per week. Throughout her life, she had travelled widely in Africa and Asia.

Examination revealed no abnormal signs and her blood tests were unremarkable.

Her plain chest X-ray is shown below.

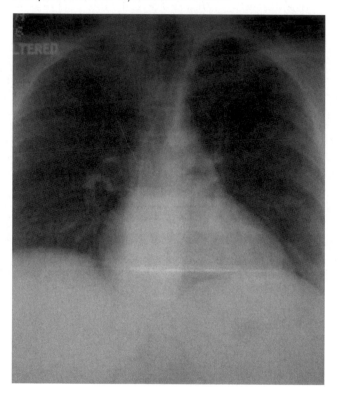

1   Which of the following is the most likely diagnosis?

- [ ] A   Tracheo-oesophageal fistula
- [ ] B   Carcinoma of the lung
- [ ] C   Achalasia
- [ ] D   Chagas' disease
- [ ] E   Pharyngeal pouch

Case 23

A 58-year-old Greek lady attended A&E with a 4-week history of discomfort in the right upper quadrant.

Examination revealed that she was mildly tender in the right upper quadrant and had 4-cm hepatomegaly. She had a previous laparotomy scar, having had a duodenal ulcer oversewn 20 years previously.

Liver function tests were normal, as was the full blood count. Her abdominal X-ray is shown below.

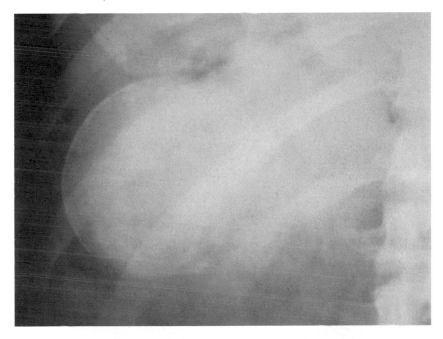

1   What is the most likely diagnosis?

- [ ] A   Porcelain gallbladder
- [ ] B   Hydatid disease
- [ ] C   Amoebic liver abscess
- [ ] D   Pyogenic liver abscess
- [ ] E   Retained foreign body from previous surgery

Case 24

A 32-year-old psychiatric patient was found to have iron deficiency anaemia on routine blood testing and was referred for an opinion. She complained of anorexia, fullness in her abdomen and, more recently, vomiting after eating solids. She was not vegetarian and said that she ate a varied diet, although she did suffer from menorrhagia. She had lost a little weight recently.

Examination revealed that she had a large mass in her upper abdomen. This was found to be non-tender, non-pulsatile and not to move on ventilation. Other than pale conjunctivae and thinning hair, no other signs were found. Her blood tests confirmed iron deficiency anaemia, but were otherwise normal.

Her plain abdominal X-ray is shown below.

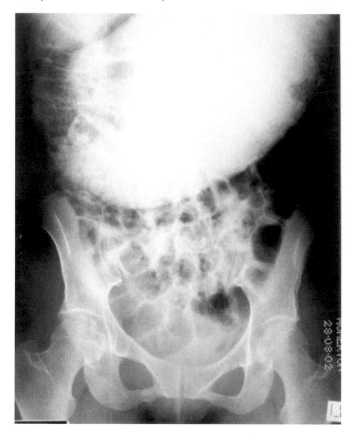

1   Which of the following is the most likely diagnosis?

- ☐ A   Bezoar
- ☐ B   Gastric carcinoma
- ☐ C   Duodenal ulcer
- ☐ D   Pancreatic carcinoma
- ☐ E   Cystocele of the gallbladder

Case 25

A 19-year-old woman presented to A&E with abdominal pain and vomiting. She had a long history of intermittent cramping abdominal pain, as did her younger brother, and her father had had two laparotomies.

Examination and investigation revealed signs of small-bowel obstruction. A picture of her mouth is shown below.

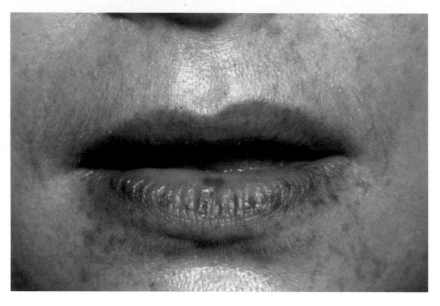

1   What is the diagnosis?

- [ ] A   Hereditary haemorrhagic telangiectasia (HHT)
- [ ] B   Juvenile polyposis
- [ ] C   Familial adenomatous polyposis (FAP)
- [ ] D   Peutz–Jegher syndrome
- [ ] E   Cronkhite–Canada syndrome

Case 26

A 55-year-old woman with a known history of coeliac disease was reviewed in Outpatients complaining of watery diarrhoea ten times per day and abdominal cramping pains of 10 months' duration. There was no accompanying weight loss. She claimed to have been adhering to her gluten-free diet and gave no history of foreign travel or changes in her medication. She took aspirin and digoxin for chronic atrial fibrillation and ibuprofen for osteoarthritis.

Examination revealed a well-looking lady who was in rate-controlled atrial fibrillation. No other abnormalities were noted.

Full blood count, electrolytes, serum calcium, immunoglobulins, CRP and the ESR were normal. IgA anti-endomysial antibodies were negative.

The colonic mucosa looked normal at colonoscopy. A biopsy specimen taken at the time is shown below.

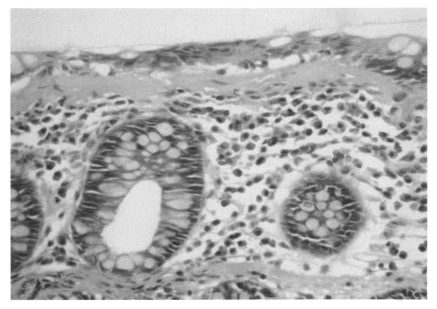

1   What is the diagnosis?

- [ ] A   Ulcerative colitis
- [ ] B   Poorly controlled coeliac disease
- [ ] C   Coeliac disease-related lymphoma
- [ ] D   Ischaemic colitis
- [ ] E   Collagenous colitis

Case 27

A 27-year-old woman recently diagnosed with inflammatory bowel disease attended A&E with severe upper abdominal pain. She also had epilepsy which was difficult to control, requiring recent manipulation of her drug therapy.

On examination she was tachycardic (110 bpm), hypotensive (95/55 mmHg) and had marked epigastric tenderness.

Blood results were as follows:

Hb	8.6 g/dL
MCV	85 fL
WCC	13.0×10^9/L
Platelets	387×10^9/L
Sodium	137 mmol/L
Potassium	4.5 mmol/L
Urea	5.4 mmol/L
Creatinine	98 mmol/L
Corrected Ca^{2+}	2.1 μmol/L
Amylase	1635 U/L

1   Which of the following drugs that she is taking is least likely to be the cause?

☐ A 6-mercaptopurine
☐ B Phenobarbital
☐ C Prednisolone
☐ D 5-aminosalicylic acid
☐ E Sodium valproate

Case 28

A 79-year-old man was referred by his GP with a 4-month history of dysphagia. He was unable to pinpoint the site of his symptoms accurately but noted that his dysphagia worsened as he ate. At times he would regurgitate food during his meals, which would temporarily relieve his symptoms. According to his GP, who had weighed him, he had lost 1 kg in weight over the past 2 months. His medications included bendroflumethiazide for hypertension and ranitidine, which he took intermittently for symptoms of gastro-oesophageal reflux disease.

A barium swallow is shown below.

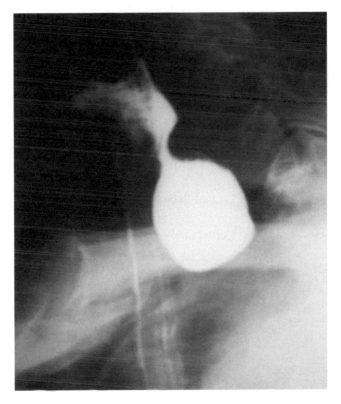

1   What is the diagnosis?

- A   Schatzki ring
- B   Achalasia
- C   Benign oesophageal stricture
- D   Pharyngeal pouch
- E   Post-cricoid web

Case 29

A 17-year-old Turkish girl presented to A&E with a 4-hour history of severe abdominal pain. The onset was rapid and without preceding symptoms. She described no change in her bowel habit or urinary symptoms. She had had an appendectomy 6 months previously and an exploratory laparotomy 2 months ago for similar episodes. At neither operation was any abnormality found other than a small amount of peritoneal fluid.

On examination she was pyrexial at 39.2 °C and tachycardic at 105 bpm. Her abdomen was diffusely tender with guarding in the right upper quadrant. Bowel sounds were reduced. A painful erythematous rash was noted on the lower limbs.

Investigations were as follows:

Urinalysis	Blood +
Hb	13.6 g/dL
MCV	85 fL
WCC	14.8×10^9/L
Platelets	387×10^9/L
CRP	55 mg/L
β-HCG	< 5 U/L
Erect chest X-ray	Normal

1   Which of the following is the most likely diagnosis?

- ☐ A   Ectopic pregnancy
- ☐ B   Recurrent polyserositis
- ☐ C   Acute intermittent porphyria
- ☐ D   Renal colic
- ☐ E   Abdominal angina

Case 30

A 27-year-old lady who was 16 weeks pregnant was referred for an opinion by the obstetricians because of recurrent vomiting. She had started vomiting early in her pregnancy and had not responded to treatment with anti-emetics. She now weighed 5kg less than when she became pregnant. Nasogastric and nasojejunal feeding were unsuccessful due to recurrent regurgitation of the tubes. Accordingly, total parenteral nutrition (TPN) was commenced. She also required supplemental intravenous fluids due to continued vomiting.

Her blood tests were checked 72 hours after initiating TPN and were as follows:

Sodium	137 mmol/L
Potassium	2.9 mmol/L
Urea	2.4 mmol/L
Creatinine	69 μmol/L
Corrected Ca^{2+}	2.2 mmol/L
Phosphate$_4$	0.2 mmol/L
Magnesium	0.4 mmol/L

1   What is the most likely explanation for these results?

- [ ] A   Bloods taken from drip arm
- [ ] B   Syndrome of inappropriate ADH secretion
- [ ] C   Inappropriate intravenous fluid replacement
- [ ] D   Refeeding syndrome
- [ ] E   Vomiting-related electrolyte loss

Case 31

A 44-year-old gentleman with a long history of diarrhoea presented with a painful lesion on his leg. He had noticed what he thought was an insect bite some days previously, which rapidly progressed to the lesion depicted. He had started feeling unwell with the development of the lesion and described general malaise and arthralgia.

A picture of the lesion and a barium enema are shown below.

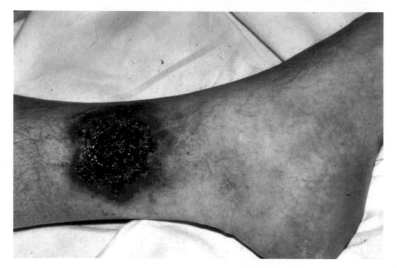

1   What two diagnoses are shown?

- [ ] A Pyoderma gangrenosum
- [ ] B Crohn's disease
- [ ] C Acanthosis nigricans
- [ ] D Ulcerative colitis
- [ ] E Ogilvie's syndrome
- [ ] F Ischaemic colitis
- [ ] G Erythema nodosum
- [ ] H Erythema multiforme
- [ ] I   Colonic carcinoma
- [ ] J Dermatomyositis

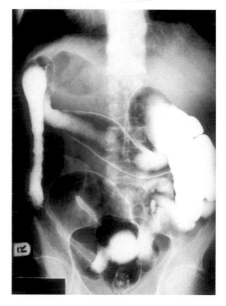

Case 32

A 55-year-old lady was admitted via A&E complaining of intermittent epigastric pain. She had had a cholecystectomy 1 year ago for these symptoms but continued to have pain after the procedure. The pain was severe, typically came on when she was eating, radiated to the back and was accompanied by nausea and sometimes vomiting. It tended to last for several hours and did not vary in intensity. She had had five attacks over the last year.

Blood results at the time of her admission are shown:

Bilirubin	21 μmol/L
AST	100 U/L
ALT	110 U/L
ALP	176 U/L
Amylase	220 U/L

An ultrasound scan showed a moderately dilated common bile duct (12 mm) but no stones were seen. Consequently, she underwent an endoscopic retrograde cholangiogram which, again, showed mildly dilated ducts. A sphincterotomy was performed along with trawling of the bile duct, again revealing no cause. Post-procedure she developed acute pancreatitis from which she recovered with conservative management. Subsequently, her symptoms resolved.

1   Which of the following is the most likely diagnosis?

- [ ] A   Recurrent biliary stones
- [ ] B   Non-ulcer dyspepsia
- [ ] C   Chronic pancreatitis
- [ ] D   Sphincter of Oddi dysfunction
- [ ] F   Primary sclerosing cholangitis

Case 33

A 56-year-old gentleman is brought to the hospital after collapsing in the street. On arrival he is alert but disorientated and smells strongly of alcohol. He complains of a sore tongue.

Examination reveals that he is unkempt and malnourished, with angular stomatitis and glossitis. A picture of his hands is shown below.

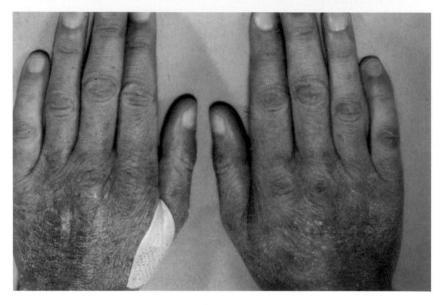

1   What are the changes on his hands most likely due to?

- A   Vitamin B$_{12}$ deficiency
- B   Vitamin C deficiency
- C   Thiamine deficiency
- D   Niacin deficiency
- E   Riboflavin deficiency

Case 34

A 55-year-old gentleman attended A&E with haematemesis half an hour previously. He was visiting the UK from Africa but had been well prior to presentation. On arrival he was shocked and pale and therefore underwent upper gastrointestinal endoscopy after adequate resuscitation.

Blood tests on arrival were as follows:

Hb	6.6 g/dL
MCV	65 fL
WCC	6.0×10^9/L
Platelets	87×10^9/L
Albumin	40 g/L
Bilirubin	5 μmol/L
AST	12 U/L
ALT	13 U/L
ALP	66 U/L
INR	1.0

Examination of the oesophagus revealed large varices with stigmata of recent bleeding. No blood was seen but two red worms, about 10 mm in length, were noted adherent to the mucosa in the duodenum.

1 Which two agents is he most likely to be infected with?

☐ A   *Trichuris trichiura*
☐ B   *Necator americanus*
☐ C   Hepatitis B virus
☐ D   *Schistosoma haematobium*
☐ E   *Strongyloides stercoralis*
☐ F   *Ascaris lumbricoides*
☐ G   Hepatitis C virus
☐ H   *Schistosoma mansoni*
☐ I   *Enterobius vermicularis*

Case 35

A 45-year-old lady attended A&E with a 4-hour history of acute severe central abdominal pain that was colicky in nature and associated with nausea and vomiting. Other than hypertension, for which she had recently started a β-blocker and an angiotensin-converting enzyme inhibitor, she was fit and well with no past medical or surgical history and no family history of note.

Her plain abdominal X-ray is shown below.

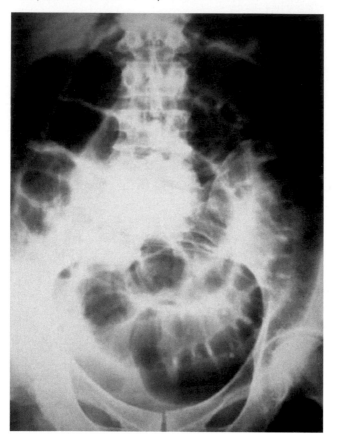

1   What is the most likely diagnosis?

- [ ] A   Ogilvie's syndrome
- [ ] B   Angio-oedema of the bowel
- [ ] C   Gallstone ileus
- [ ] D   Adhesions
- [ ] E   Irritable bowel syndrome

Case 36

A 42-year-old man presented to his GP complaining of lethargy, pruritus, right upper quadrant discomfort and dry mouth and eyes. Otherwise he was asymptomatic and had no previous history of note. He drank 24 units of alcohol per week.

On examination, he had two-finger hepatomegaly and his spleen was just palpable. No signs of chronic liver disease were present.

Blood tests were as follows:

Sodium	132 mmol/L
Potassium	4.4 mmol/L
Urea	2.4 mmol/L
Creatinine	70 μmol/L
Albumin	34 g/L
Bilirubin	25 μmol/L
AST	44 U/L
ALT	41 U/L
ALP	556 U/L
GGT	1021 U/L
Serum LDL cholesterol	3.22 mmol/L
Serum HDL cholesterol	5.56 mmol/L
Serum IgM	6.5 g/L

1   What is the most likely diagnosis?

- A   Gallstones
- B   Pancreatic carcinoma
- C   Primary sclerosing cholangitis (PSC)
- D   Primary biliary cirrhosis (PBC)
- E   Haemochromatosis

Case 37

A 65-year-old woman is brought to A&E by her husband, complaining of upper abdominal and lower chest pain radiating to the back. As part of their fortieth wedding anniversary celebrations, they had been out for a large meal at which they had consumed more alcohol than they were normally used to. On returning home, she had become nauseated and had vomited three times. Concurrently, she developed upper abdominal and lower chest pain and, subsequently, shortness of breath.

On examination, she was tachycardic at 105 bpm, tachypnoeic at 25 breaths per minute and was pyrexial at 37.8 °C. She had firmness in the upper abdomen and a plain chest X-ray confirmed the clinical findings of a left pleural effusion.

1 Which of the following is the most likely diagnosis?

☐ A Mallory–Weiss tear
☐ B Spontaneous pneumothorax
☐ C Acute pancreatitis
☐ D Perforated peptic ulcer
☐ E Boerhaave syndrome

Case 38

A 67-year-old gentleman of Irish descent presented to Outpatients with a 10-month history of right iliac fossa abdominal pain and watery diarrhoea up to 15 times a day. He had been a heavy drinker in the past, consuming 40 pints of beer a week, but had cut back to 1 pint a day for several years. He had recently noticed that his symptoms became worse when he drank alcohol and so had now stopped completely. His wife had noticed that he had lost weight recently but he was unable to quantify this. He had never smoked but his wife had noticed that he had had some attacks of wheeziness.

Examination of his abdomen revealed 3-cm hepatomegaly and an indistinct mass in the right iliac fossa. Urea and electrolytes, liver function tests and full blood count were normal, but a small-bowel barium examination revealed a submucosal mass in the ileum.

1   What is the likely diagnosis?

- ☐ A   Coeliac disease-related lymphoma
- ☐ B   Chronic pancreatitis
- ☐ C   Villous adenoma
- ☐ D   Carcinoid syndrome
- ☐ E   Immunoproliferative small intestinal disease (IPSID)

Case 39

A 44-year-old woman attended A&E complaining of shortness of breath and tiredness. She had recently started oral treatment for an intensely itchy, vesicular rash on the elbows, knees, buttocks and back. She also gave a history of mild diarrhoea and abdominal bloating, and had lost a stone in weight.

Her blood results were as follows (RDW, red cell distribution width):

Hb	5.6 g/dL
MCV	90 fL
WCC	5.8×10^9/L
Platelets	387×10^9/L
RDW	22%
Sodium	138 mmol/L
Potassium	4.4 mmol/L
Urea	4.4 mmol/L
Creatinine	99 μmol/L
Albumin	32 g/L
Corrected Ca^{2+}	2.0 mmol/L
Bilirubin	30 μmol/L

1 **Which two of the following are most likely to be contributing to her anaemia?**

- [ ] A Autoimmune haemolysis
- [ ] B Drug-related haemolysis
- [ ] C Iron deficiency due to malabsorption
- [ ] D Vitamin B_{12} deficiency
- [ ] E Anaemia of chronic disease
- [ ] F Gastrointestinal blood loss
- [ ] G Bone marrow suppression
- [ ] H Sideroblastic anaemia

Case 40

A 47-year-old woman attends Outpatients asking for advice. She has a family history of colorectal carcinoma. Her family tree is shown below (patient arrowed).

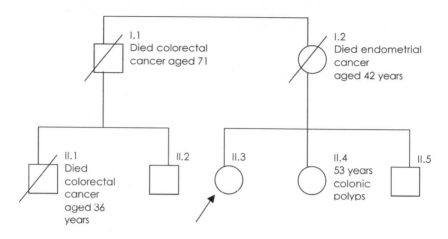

1   What is the most likely explanation for the family's history?

☐   A   Familial adenomatous polyposis (FAP)
☐   B   Hereditary non-polyposis colorectal cancer
☐   C   Sporadic colorectal carcinoma
☐   D   Peutz–Jegher syndrome
☐   E   Attenuated familial adenomatous polyposis

Case 41

A 69-year-old gentleman presented to A&E claiming to have swallowed a foreign object 2 hours previously. He had a long history of mental health problems and had presented with a similar history in the past. He denied any dysphagia, odynophagia or abdominal pain, and physical examination was unremarkable.

His plain abdominal X-ray is shown below.

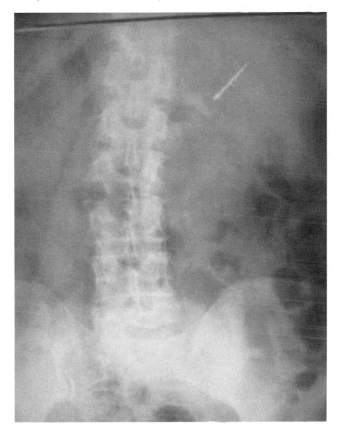

1   What course of action would you advise?

- [ ] A   Laparotomy and removal of the object
- [ ] B   Endoscopic removal of the object
- [ ] C   Reassure and discharge the patient
- [ ] D   Monitor with weekly X-rays to ensure passage through the gastrointestinal tract
- [ ] E   Metoclopramide or other gastrointestinal stimulants

Chapter Four

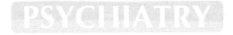

Case 1

A 52-year-old homeless alcoholic man presented to A&E with a 2-week history of general malaise, abulia, insomnia and worsening anorexia. For the last 3 days he had been unable to tolerate alcohol. He also described recent headache, sweating and palpitations. His GP had prescribed paroxetine 6 months earlier for depression without benefit, and he now presented severely depressed and suicidal.

Physical examination revealed signs of chronic liver disease. Sensation to pinprick and light touch was reduced in a stocking distribution and his leg muscles were painful and tender. Tone was mildly raised in the lower limbs and the reflexes were symmetrically brisk, except at the ankles where they were absent. Urine drug screen was negative and paracetamol and salicylate were undetectable. His blood results were:

Hb	11.9 g/dL
MCV	103 fL
WCC	4.5×10^9/L
Platelets	105×10^9/L
ALT	74 U/L
Albumin	32 g/L
Sodium	129 mmol/L
Urea	3.1 mmol/L

1   What is the most likely diagnosis?

- [ ] A   Wernicke–Korsakoff syndrome
- [ ] B   Alcoholic hallucinosis
- [ ] C   Central pontine myelinolysis
- [ ] D   Pellagra
- [ ] E   Paroxetine overdose
- [ ] F   Paroxetine discontinuation syndrome
- [ ] G   Subdural haematoma
- [ ] H   Delirium tremens
- [ ] I   Chronic alcohol dependency
- [ ] J   Korsakoff's syndrome

He was admitted to an acute psychiatric ward and nursed one-to-one because of ongoing suicidal ideation. Four days after starting on chlordiazepoxide detoxification he became increasingly disorientated and confused and was seen responding to auditory hallucinations. He became convinced that the nurse with him planned to murder him in his sleep. He was incontinent of urine and faeces. On repeat examination he was found to be ataxic with extrapyramidal rigidity.

2   What additional diagnosis/complication has occurred?

☐ A   Wernicke–Korsakoff syndrome
☐ B   Alcoholic hallucinosis
☐ C   Central pontine myelinolysis
☐ D   Pellagra
☐ E   Paroxetine overdose
☐ F   Paroxetine discontinuation syndrome
☐ G   Subdural haematoma
☐ H   Delirium tremens
☐ I   Chronic alcohol dependency
☐ J   Korsakoff's syndrome

3   What treatment should be instigated immediately?

☐ A   Pabrinex®
☐ B   Chlordiazepoxide
☐ C   Haloperidol intramuscularly
☐ D   Clonidine
☐ E   Thiamine intravenously
☐ F   Olanzapine 10 mg
☐ G   Neurosurgical referral

Case 2

A 23-year-old Swedish student was brought to A&E by her boyfriend who was concerned that she had been acting strangely for 48 hours. She had become increasingly agitated and restless, claiming that her flatmate was monitoring her behaviour and trying to steal her identity. She had not slept for 2 nights. On two occasions she had become unresponsive, staring blankly ahead, following which she appeared confused and disorientated. She had vomited twice and was complaining of severe abdominal pain that she ascribed to menstruation. She had had two similar though less severe episodes around the time of menstruation in the last 2 months. She had been well until 6 months previously, when she had became depressed at the time of her end-of-year exams and had been prescribed fluvoxamine by her GP.

On examination she appeared confused and was disorientated to time. Abdominal examination revealed central tenderness without guarding. Other than sinus tachycardia, the respiratory and cardiovascular examinations were unremarkable. Neurological exam revealed reduced sensation distally and reduced power on shoulder abduction bilaterally.

Some investigations are performed:

Hb	12.8 g/dL
WCC	11.0×10^9/L
Sodium	127 mmol/L
Potassium	3.8 mmol/L
Urea	4.1 mmol/L
Chest X-ray	Normal
CT brain	Unremarkable

A lumbar puncture is performed:

Opening pressure	15 cmH$_2$O
RBC	2 cells/mL
WCC	4 cells/mL (all lymphocytes)
Protein	52 mg/L

1   What two things should you do?

☐ A Psychiatric referral
☐ B EEG
☐ C Toxicology screen
☐ D Urinary porphyrins

☐ E Amylase
☐ F Abdominal ultrasound
☐ G Gynaecology referral
☐ H Abdominal X-ray

2   What is the likely diagnosis?

- ☐ A   Guillain–Barré syndrome
- ☐ B   Cycloid psychosis
- ☐ C   Pre-menstrual tension
- ☐ D   Non-convulsive status epilepticus
- ☐ E   Acute intermittent porphyria (AIP)
- ☐ F   Methylenedioxymethamphetamine (MDMA, Ecstasy) toxicity

Case 3

A 32-year-old man presents to A&E with his mother, who is concerned because he has become increasingly confused and agitated. He was incontinent of urine before she called the ambulance. He is unable to give a history and appears disorientated. His mother says that he has recently seen a psychiatrist who has prescribed aripiprazole.

On examination he appears sweaty; temperature is 38.6 °C. He is tachycardic at 132 bpm and his blood pressure is 180/105 mmHg. Neurological examination reveals symmetrically raised tone in all four limbs; the plantars are bilaterally down-going. Pupillary light reflexes are normal. The investigations show:

Hb	13.6 g/dL
WCC	12.4 × 10⁹/L
Neutrophils	9.1 × 10⁹/L
Lymphocytes	2.0 × 10⁹/L
Platelets	155 × 10⁹/L
Sodium	135 mmol/L
Urea	7.8 mmol/L
Creatinine	99 μmol/L
ALT	78 U/L
γGT	299 U/L

1   What is the most likely diagnosis?

☐ A Catatonic schizophrenia
☐ B MDMA (Ecstasy) toxicity
☐ C Parasagittal meningioma
☐ D Neuroleptic malignant syndrome
☐ E Serotonin syndrome
☐ F Delirium tremens
☐ G Tardive dyskinesia
☐ H Acute dystonic reaction

2   What is the next investigation that you would perform?

☐ A Psychiatry referral
☐ B CT brain
☐ C Lumbar puncture
☐ D Creatine kinase
☐ E Urine drug screen
☐ F Blood culture

3   Which two treatments are most appropriate?

- [ ] A Lorazepam
- [ ] B Intramuscular haloperidol
- [ ] C Dantrolene
- [ ] D Procyclidine
- [ ] E Naloxone
- [ ] F Bromocriptine
- [ ] G Neurosurgical referral

Case 4

A 36-year old artist presented to A&E with a friend who was concerned that she had been acting strangely and had appeared intermittently confused over the last 3 days. She said that she had been feeling increasingly anxious and restless over the last week and had been to the health food store to buy some St John's wort to pick her up. Her only other medication is venlafaxine prescribed by her GP. For 2 days she had been feeling nauseated and had developed diarrhoea.

On examination she was mildly disorientated in time, was shivering and appeared restless. She was tachycardic at 120 bpm and her blood pressure was raised at 150/95 mmHg. Temperature was 37.6 °C. Neurological examination revealed a fine tremor in the upper limbs and multifocal myoclonus. Reflexes were symmetrically brisk, plantars down-going. There was no neck stiffness. Blood tests were unremarkable.

1   What is the most likely diagnosis?

- [ ] A   Neuroleptic malignant syndrome
- [ ] B   Serotonin syndrome
- [ ] C   Delirium tremens
- [ ] D   Tardive dyskinesia
- [ ] E   Akathisia
- [ ] F   SSRI discontinuation syndrome
- [ ] G   New variant CJD

Chapter Five

RENAL MEDICINE

Case 1

A 30-year-old gentleman with a 12-year history of AIDS, with a good response to therapy, was admitted with a 12-day history of weakness, nausea, dysuria, myalgia and decreased urine output. His last CD4 lymphocyte count was 368 × 10⁶/L (normal range 500–900). The current medications included didanosine, stavudine, atorvastatin, trimethoprim-sulfamethoxazole, and he had been commenced on indinavir.

On examination he was afebrile, pulse 100 bpm and regular, BP 176/99 mmHg, the JVP was not elevated; the chest and abdominal examinations were normal.

Investigations:

Hb	13.5 g/dL
WCC	6.7 × 10⁹/L
Platelets	200 × 10⁹/L
Sodium	135 mmol/L
Potassium	5.2 mmol/L
Chloride	102 mmol/L
Bicarbonate	16 mmol/L
Urea	29.2 mmol/L
Creatinine	765 µmol/L
Bone profile	Normal
Creatine kinase	100 U/L
ANCA	Negative
Anti-GBM	Negative
Hep B/hep C	Negative
ASOT	Negative

Cultures of blood/urine/sputum were negative.

1   Which one of the following medications is the most likely cause of his acute renal failure?

☐   A   Didanosine
☐   B   Stavudine
☐   C   Indinavir
☐   D   Atorvastatin
☐   E   Trimethoprin-sulfamethoxazole

2   Which of the following investigations will be most helpful in making the diagnosis?

☐   A   Native renal biopsy
☐   B   Renal ultrasound scan
☐   C   Urine for crystals
☐   D   X-ray studies of kidneys, ureters, bladder (KUB)
☐   E   Serum immunoglobulins

Case 2

A 28-year-old Somalian lady presented to A&E with a 3-week history of generalised weakness, anorexia, decreased appetite, and weight loss. She was noted to be increasingly short of breath and had intermittent headaches. She worked as a cleaner and has been in the UK for 3 years. She was unable to give a sexual history. There was no history of blood transfusions.

On examination she appeared cachectic, afebrile, pulse 80 bpm and regular, BP 130/80 mmHg, JVP not seen. There was no peripheral oedema. Chest examination was normal. Fundoscopy revealed grade 2 hypertensive retinopathy. The remainder of examination was normal.

Investigations:

Hb	9.2 g/dL
WCC	4.1×10^9/L
Platelets	100×10^9/L
Blood film	Microcytosis
Sodium	138 mmol/L
Potassium	3.2 mmol/L
Urea	18 mmol/L
Creatinine	205 µmol/L
Total protein	58 g/L
Albumin	18 g/L
LFTs	Normal
Bone profile	Normal
Urine microscopy	Intact red blood cells/granular casts
Blood/urine culture	Negative
CXR	Normal
ECG	Normal
Renal ultrasound scan	Highly echogenic kidneys Right kidney 13.5 cm; left kidney 14 cm

She underwent a native renal biopsy.

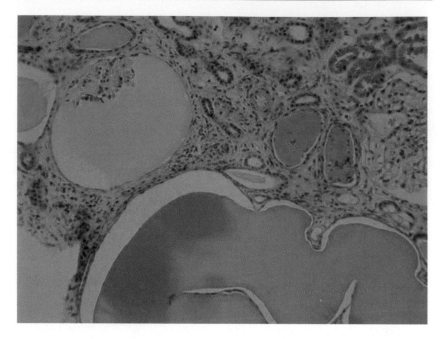

1   What is most likely diagnosis?

☐   A   Primary focal segmental glomerulosclerosis
☐   B   Schistosomiasis
☐   C   HIV-associated nephropathy (HIVAN)
☐   D   Heroin-associated nephropathy
☐   E   Malignant hypertension

Case 3

A 70 year-old white man with a history of intermittent microscopic haematuria presented with generalised fatigue, cough, and vague abdominal pain and diarrhoea. He has a history of hypertension and was on irbesartan. Baseline renal function was normal when checked by his GP 3 weeks previously.

Initial investigations:

Hb	7.8 g/dL
Haematocrit	0.4
Platelets	98×10^6/mL
Creatinine	250 μmol/L
Amylase	150 U/L
LFTs	Normal

Urine microscopy was not done on admission.

Ultrasound scans of abdomen and pelvis were normal.

The chest radiograph is as below.

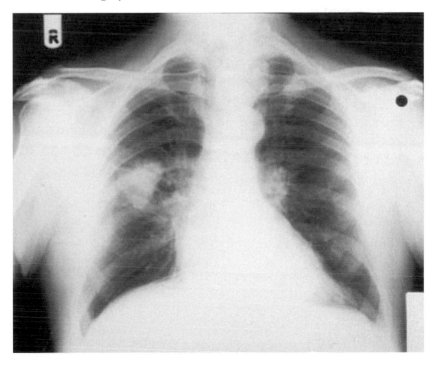

He was treated with ciprofloxacin for a presumed chest infection. He then developed acute ischaemic bowel requiring resection, with non-specific pathological findings. The hospital course was complicated by hypotension and multi-organ failure. The creatinine rose to 636 µmol/L with anuria; haemodialysis was initiated.

Urine microscopy	Numerous red blood cells
Protein excretion	3 g/24 h
ANA, ANCA	Negative
HBsAg	Negative
HCV	Negative
Cryoglobulins	Negative
C_3	107 mg/dL (NR 65–190 mg/dL)
C_4	38 mg/dL (NR 15–50 mg/dL)
Protein electrophoresis	Normal pattern

Renal biopsy was performed which showed crescentic glomerulonephritis with linear IgG staining on immunofluorescence.

1   What is the most likely diagnosis?

- [ ] A Post-streptococcal glomerulonephritis
- [ ] B Haemolytic uraemic syndrome
- [ ] C Acute pyelonephritis
- [ ] D Microscopic polyangiitis
- [ ] E Anti-glomerular basement membrane disease

Case 4

A 28-year-old man with Alport's syndrome received a pre-emptive living related renal transplant from his mother. He has excellent primary graft function and the baseline creatinine was 102 μmol/L. Three months later he presented with a 1-week history of decreased urine output with a raised creatinine of 188 μmol/L; the biopsy did not show evidence of acute rejection.

Urine microscopy showed dysmorphic red blood cells. He became progressively oligo-anuric and became dialysis-dependent.

1   What is the most likely diagnosis?

- ☐   A   Anti-glomerular basement membrane disease
- ☐   B   *Aspergillus* pneumonia
- ☐   C   Post-transplant lymphoproliferative disorder
- ☐   D   *Mycoplasma* pneumonia
- ☐   E   Wegener's granulomatosis

Case 5

A 33-year-old white man was admitted with a 1-week history of rash, pyrexia, generalised weakness and decreased urine output.

On examination he was obese, with a temperature of 38.5 °C, BP 156/70 mmHg. He had nail-fold vasculitic skin lesions. On auscultation he had a soft systolic murmur. Abdominal examination was limited given his size, but unremarkable.

Initial investigations revealed:

Hb	9 g/dL
WCC	18.5×10^9/L
Neutrophils	16.4×10^9/L
Platelets	80×10^9/L
Creatinine	336 μmol/L

Urine microscopy	Red cell casts
Hepatitis B	Negative
Hepatitis C	Negative
ANCA/GBM	Negative
Cryoglobulins	Positive
ASOT	Negative
Protein electrophoresis	Negative

Ultrasound scan of the abdomen showed an 11-cm spleen.

Renal biopsy was not performed, as it was not technically possible.

1   What is the most likely diagnosis?

- ☐ A   Microscopic polyangiitis
- ☐ B   Infective endocarditis
- ☐ C   Acute pyelonephritis
- ☐ D   HIV-associated nephropathy (HIVAN)
- ☐ E   Renal tuberculosis

Case 6

A 50-year-old man presented with a 4-month history of hypertension, headaches, and impaired vision. Two weeks ago he noted blood in his urine. His medical history was significant – he had a left nephrectomy 16 years previously.

The following is the MRI scan of his abdomen and brain:

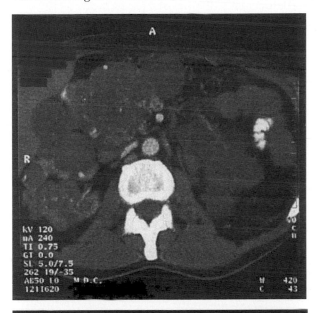

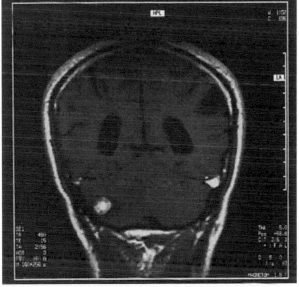

131

1   What is the diagnosis?

☐   A   Autosomal dominant polycystic kidney disease (ADPKD)
☐   B   Autosomal recessive polycystic kidney disease (ARPKD)
☐   C   Tuberose sclerosis (TSC)
☐   D   von Hippel–Lindau disease
☐   E   Histiocytosis X

Case 7

A 50-year-old white woman presented to her GP with a 2-week history of nausea, vomiting, and anorexia. She had mild epistaxis and scant haemoptysis for the last 6 to 8 months, with three episodes of sinusitis, treated with antibiotics and inhaled steroids. Her serum creatinine on presentation was 144 µmol/L with protein 1+ and blood+++. Urine microscopy revealed granular casts and dysmorphic red blood cells. She was referred to the hospital medical team the next day when her creatinine was 175 µmol/L.

The blood pressure was 160/98 mmHg, with no rashes or other findings on physical examination.

Investigations:

Creatinine	256 µmol/L
Haematocrit	0.36
Platelets	300×10^9/L
WCC	6.1×10^9/L
ANA	Negative
C_3	71 mg/dL (NR 65–190 mg/dL)
C_4	37 mg/dL (NR 15–50 mg/dL)

1   What is the most likely diagnosis?

☐ A   pANCA-positive vasculitis
☐ B   cANCA-positive vasculitis
☐ C   Lupus nephritis
☐ D   Post-streptococcal glomerulonephritis
☐ E   Henoch–Schönlein purpura (HSP)

Case 8

A 72-year-old Bangladeshi gentleman with a new diagnosis of type 2 diabetes, presented with a 3-week history of leg oedema. His past medical history includes hospitalisation after a road traffic accident 20 years ago in Bangladesh and stable angina. There was no history of retinopathy or neuropathy. Current medications include aspirin 75 mg, atorvastatin 20 mg, amlodipine 5 mg once daily, and isosorbide mononitrate SR 60 mg once a day. His diabetic control with dietary modification has been satisfactory with an HbA$_{1c}$ of 6.2%.

Investigations:

Creatinine	68 μmol/L
Bilirubin	5 μmol/L
ALT	30 U/L
ALP	98 U/L
γGT	45 U/L
Total protein	32 g/L
Albumin	18 g/L
Cholesterol	9.8 mmol/L
Urine microscopy	Granular casts
Urine protein	14.2 g/day

Hepatitis serology:

B e antigen	Negative
B core IgG antibody	Positive
B surface antigen	Positive
C antibody	Negative

Renal biopsy was performed and is shown opposite.

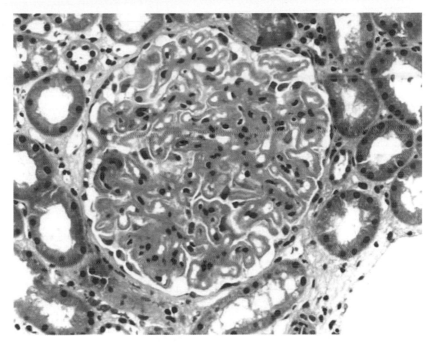

1   What is the most likely diagnosis?

☐ A   Renal TB
☐ B   Mesangiocapillary glomerulonephritis (MCGN)
☐ C   Minimal-change disease
☐ D   Diabetic glomerulosclerosis
☐ E   Membranous nephropathy

Case 9

A 68-year-old Ghanaian gentleman with a 10-year history of type 2 diabetes presented with a 3-week history of generalised oedema. In spite of insulin treatment, his diabetes has been poorly controlled. He has background retinopathy. Investigations revealed normal renal function; albumin 12 g/L; negative ANA, ANCA, GBM, HBsAg, hepatitis C antibody, cryoglobulins and serum electrophoresis; 24-hour urine protein excretion was 15.6 g.

He underwent a renal biopsy.

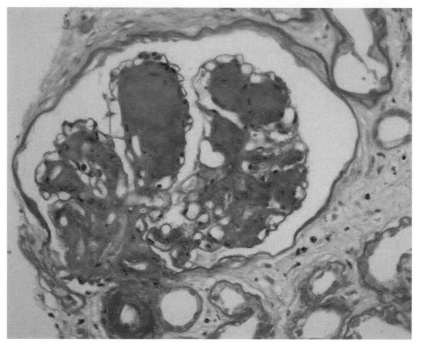

1   What is the most likely diagnosis?

☐   A   Focal segmental glomerulosclerosis
☐   B   Membranous nephropathy
☐   C   Light-chain disease
☐   D   Diabetic glomerulosclerosis
☐   E   Minimal change disease

Case 10

A 19-year-old man presented with a 2-day history of a painful rash, constipation, lethargy and generalised body pain. He has no significant past medical history apart from hospitalisation as child for peritonitis secondary to a ruptured appendix.

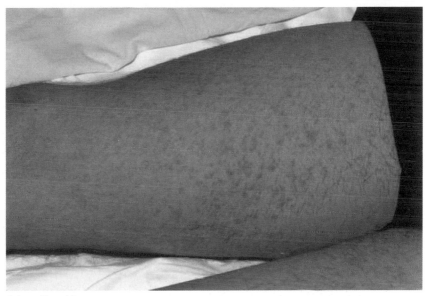

Science Photo Library

Investigations:

Creatinine	162 µmol/l
LFTs	Normal
FBC	Normal
Urine microscopy	Red cell casts
ANCA	Negative
ASOT	Normal
Hepatitis B/C	Negative

1   What is the diagnosis?

- ☐ A   IgA nephropathy
- ☐ B   Infective endocarditis
- ☐ C   Henoch–Schönlein purpura (HSP)
- ☐ D   Erythema nodosum
- ☐ E   Polyarteritis nodosa

Case 11

A 24-year-old South Asian woman presented with acute onset of left-sided flank pain with microscopic haematuria. She had a KUB X-ray performed. She has a history of recurrent urinary tract infections since childhood and in the past was investigated and treated by a urology specialist. Her maternal first cousin is on peritoneal dialysis for end-stage renal disease.

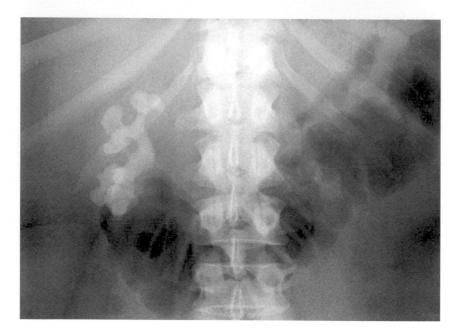

Her investigations:

Creatinine	96 µmol/L
Calcium	2.48 mmol/L
Phosphate	1.02 mmol/L
Albumin	40 g/L
Urine protein	0.5 g/24 h
Creatinine clearance	68 mL/minute
24-h urine calcium	10 mmol (NR < 7.5 mmol)
24-h urine oxalate	1.4 mmol (NR < 0.36 mmol)
24-h urine urate	3.2 mmol (NR < 4.5 mmol)

1   What is the most likely diagnosis?

- [ ] A   Primary hyperoxaluria
- [ ] B   Primary hyperparathyroidism
- [ ] C   Secondary hyperparathyroidism
- [ ] D   Nephrogenic diabetes insipidus
- [ ] E   Surreptitious antacid ingestion

Case 12

A 37-year-old woman presents with a 2-week history of malaise, bruising, and altered bowel habit. She has no past medical history of note and is on no medications. Systemic examination is unremarkable. Urine output for the past 2 hours was 180 mL.

Investigations:

Hb	6.2 g/dL
Haematocrit	0.24
Platelets	56 × 10⁹/L
Blood film	Fragmented red cells
Urea	14 mmol/L
Creatinine	236 µmol/L

1   What is the best treatment option?

- ☐ A   Transfusion with packed red cells to aim for a haemoglobin of 10 g/dL
- ☐ B   Intravenous vitamin K
- ☐ C   Intravenous tranexamic acid
- ☐ D   Intravenous fresh frozen plasma
- ☐ E   Haemodialysis

Case 13

A 44-year-old man has been referred to the nephrologists with a serum creatinine of 210 µmol/L. He has a 15-year history of osteoarthritis . One year ago he was diagnosed with diabetes mellitus and essential hypertension. His current medications include ramipril 10 mg, aspirin 75 mg, diclofenac 150 mg and atorvastatin 10 mg daily.

On examination his BP was 110/70. Systemic examination was normal.

Investigations:

Hb	10.9 g/dL
WCC	7.2×10^9/L
Platelets	210×10^9/L
Sodium	138 mmol/L
Potassium	4.2 mmol/L
Urea	14.2 mmol/L
Creatinine	224 µmol/L
Calcium	2.28 mmol/L
Phosphate	1.05 mmol/L
Albumin	38 g/L
HbA$_{1c}$	5.5%
ECG	Normal
Urine protein	0.9 g/24 h
Renal ultrasound scan	Unobstructed echogenic kidneys
	Right kidney 9.4 cm; left kidney 8.8 cm

1   What is the most likely cause of his renal impairment?

- [ ] A   Renovascular disease
- [ ] B   Hypertensive nephrosclerosis
- [ ] C   Analgesic nephropathy
- [ ] D   Herbal nephropathy
- [ ] E   Diabetic nephropathy

Case 14

A 66-year-old gentleman on peritoneal dialysis for end-stage renal failure presents with a 3-month history of tiredness secondary to anaemia, in spite of increased subcutaneous erythropoietin (EPO) therapy.

Investigations:

Hb	6.2 g/dL
WCC	6.2 × 10⁹/L
Differential WCC	Normal
Platelets	200 × 10⁹/L
Haematocrit	0.2
MCV	80 fL
Reticulocyte count	0%

Faecal occult bloods	Negative
Colonoscopy	Normal
Upper gastrointestinal endoscopy	Normal
Haptoglobins	Normal

1   What is the most likely cause of his anaemia?

- ☐ A   Hypothyroidism
- ☐ B   Myelodysplasia
- ☐ C   Myelofibrosis
- ☐ D   Pure red cell aplasia
- ☐ E   Chronic lymphocytic leukaemia

Case 15

A 34-year-old gentleman with chronic renal failure is seen in the Nephrology Clinic. He is asymptomatic. His current medications include atenolol 100 mg once daily, ramipril 10 mg once daily, alfacalcidol 0.25 micrograms once daily, Calcichew® 1 tablet with meals and a multivitamin preparation.

Investigations:

Hb	9 g/dL
Haematocrit	0.3
MCV	80 fL
Urea	21 mmol/L
Creatinine	423 μmol/L
PTH	8.5 pmol/L
Ferritin	14 μg/L

1   How will you next treat his anaemia?

- ☐ A   Oral ferrous sulphate
- ☐ B   Intravenous iron
- ☐ C   Intravenous erythropoietin
- ☐ D   Red cell transfusion
- ☐ E   Subcutaneous erythropoietin

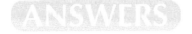

Chapter One   Answers

DERMATOLOGY

Case 1

1   B   Hypocalcaemia

This patient has lupus pernio, a cutaneous feature of sarcoidosis. Lupus pernio causes violaceous infiltrated nodules and plaques, usually on the nose. There may be associated swelling and ulceration and crusting of the nasal vestibule.

Cutaneous features of sarcoidosis can be classified as acute, subacute or chronic:

- Acute changes:
    erythema nodosum
    papular eruption
    scar sarcoid – sarcoid localises to previous sites of trauma
- Subacute changes:
    annular sarcoid
    nodular sarcoid
    angiolupoid sarcoid – rare; usually occurs in women; periorbital, soft, domed, orange-red swellings
- Chronic changes:
    plaque sarcoid
    lupus pernio
    scarring alopecia.

Lupus pernio tends to be associated with other forms of chronic fibrotic sarcoidosis. These include:

- Bone cysts – radiolucent, usually in the hands and feet
- Chronic polyarthritis – usually involving the small bones of the hands and feet
- Respiratory tract sarcoidosis – classically this causes a restrictive pattern on pulmonary function tests
- Lacrimal gland swelling – Mikulicz syndrome, ie bilateral swelling of the lacrimal and salivary glands. Sarcoid is one cause of this
- Renal sarcoid
- Hypercalcaemia.

Case 2

1   A   Discoid lupus erythematosus

This is a picture of scarring alopecia.

Alopecia can either be scarring or non-scarring, and focal or diffuse. Scarring alopecia is characterised by permanent hair loss with loss of the follicular orifices.

Causes of scarring alopecia are:

- Discoid lupus erythematosus
- Lichen planopilaris – a subtype of lichen planus. The patient often has typical lesions of lichen planus – itchy, papules over the volar aspect of the wrists with white streaks over the buccal mucosa and nail pitting
- Sarcoidosis
- Dissecting cellulitis of the scalp – classically occurs in young black men. This causes nodules and alopecia over the occiput. Ingrowing hairs and clipping the hair very short are thought to exacerbate this condition
- Follicular mucinosis – associated with cutaneous T-cell lymphoma.

Causes of a focal non-scarring alopecia are:

- Tinea capitis – scalp ringworm. Common in young children. The scalp is often scaly too
- Alopecia areata – an autoimmune disorder; associated with an increased incidence of vitiligo and thyroid disease. It typically causes patchy hair loss with 'exclamation mark hairs' at the periphery – these are formed by hairs that fracture at the distal end and taper and lose pigment proximally, so look like an exclamation mark. Usually it is restricted to the scalp but may affect any site of body hair. There is often spontaneous regrowth
- Trichotillomania – pulling of hair or use of traction in styling.

Causes of a diffuse non-scarring alopecia are:

- Androgenetic alopecia – inherited tendency. Androgen-dependent. Men are affected more than women; in women it is a rare but important allusion to the possibility of an androgen-secreting tumour. The typical pattern of thinning is at the frontal regions and crown
- Telogen effluvium – often follows major illness, stress or operation, and will regrow
- Hypo- or hyperthyroidism
- Iron deficiency
- Zinc deficiency
- Some oral contraceptive pills
- Pregnancy.

Case 3

1   **D**   Pernicious anaemia

This is vitiligo an acquired disorder of depigmentation characterised by loss of melanocytes from the epidermis. It typically presents as a hypopigmented patch with a sharp border. It often spreads to involve the body symmetrically. The pathogenesis is uncertain although there is an association with autoimmune disease and this is thought to be relevant.

A number of conditions occur in association with vitiligo. These include:

- Thyroid disease – Graves' disease (hyper-, hypo- or euthyroid), atrophic thyroid failure and Hashimoto's thyroiditis
- Type 1 diabetes mellitus
- Addison's disease
- Pernicious anaemia
- Myasthenia gravis
- Hypoparathyroidism
- Alopecia areata
- Morphoea.

Treatment of vitiligo is unsatisfactory. Some cases spontaneously resolve. Treatment with potent topical corticosteroids or PUVA phototherapy helps some.

Other causes of a depigmented patch include:

- Tinea corporis – usually overlying fine scale, post-inflammatory pigmentation, border less distinct
- Hypopigmented mycosis fungoides – cutaneous T-cell lymphoma (but one would see multiple patches and usually on the trunk)
- Leprosy

Case 4

1   B   Bendroflumethiazide

This is the distribution of a photosensitive drug eruption. The most common photosensitising drugs are:

- Thiazide diuretics
- Phenothiazines – eg chlorpromazine, promethazine
- Sulphonamides
- Oral hypoglycaemics – tolbutamide, chlorpropamide
- Tetracyclines
- Griseofulvin
- Amiodarone – chronic use leads to slate-grey pigmentation.

Beta-blockers, lithium and NSAIDs may exacerbate psoriasis. Codeine phosphate can cause a fixed drug eruption. This is a round itchy erythematous oedematous patch, with or without blistering, which fades to leave a brown discoloration of the skin. Re-challenge with the drug will cause the rash to recur in the same place. Other drugs which commonly cause a fixed drug eruption are:

- Barbiturates
- Sulphonamides
- Tetracyclines
- Salicylates
- NSAIDs.

Phenytoin commonly causes a drug rash. It is a frequent cause of erythema multiforme. In addition, it may cause the phenytoin hypersensitivity syndrome. This is characterised by a rash (often non-specific or morbilliform), fever, lymphadenopathy, hepatomegaly, eosinophilia and abnormal LFTs. Phenytoin hypersensitivity can be fatal, and there is cross-reactivity with carbamazepine, gabapentin and phenobarbital. The only 'safe' anti-epileptic drug to use in this situation is sodium valproate. In addition, first-degree relatives have a higher chance of developing the syndrome with these drugs.

Case 5

1   **A** Phenytoin treatment

This is a fissured/scrotal tongue. It is associated with:

- Geographical tongue – common and a normal variant. It affects 1% of the population; 50% also have a fissured tongue
- Granulomatous infiltration:
    Sarcoid
    Crohn's disease
    Melkersson–Rosenthal syndrome – triad of labial oedema, fissured
        tongue and recurrent unilateral facial palsy
    Trisomy 21.

Phenytoin and ciclosporin characteristically cause gingival hyperplasia.

Case 6

1   **E** *Ankylostoma braziliense*

This is a picture of cutaneous larva migrans. This is a self-limiting cutaneous eruption caused by the larvae of roundworms. *Ankylostoma braziliense* is the most common agent. Cutaneous larva migrans has a worldwide distribution but is especially prevalent in Central and Southern America. Dogs and cats carry the roundworm. Beaches are a common reservoir.

Eggs are passed in the faeces of infected animals and then hatch in soil or sand. The larvae easily penetrate skin, often causing a non-specific itchy dermatitis at the time. Migration of larvae usually occurs within a week, with the production of a wandering, thread-like, intensely pruritic, erythematous track. The larvae travel at a speed of a few mm to 2 cm daily.

The cutaneous eruption can be accompanied by breathlessness, transient pulmonary infiltrates, fever and eosinophilia – Loeffler's syndrome.

Treatment is with ivermectin 12 mg stat or albendazole 400 mg/day for 3 days.

Strongyloides stercoralis causes larva currens. Although this has a similar appearance, it migrates through the skin at a much faster rate – up to 10 cm/hour.

Toxocara canis causes toxocariasis – visceral larva migrans. Cutaneous manifestations include generalised pruritus and urticaria. Other features are eosinophilia, cough, breathlessness, muscle pains and hepatomegaly.

Sarcoptes scabei is the mite which causes scabies. Scabies is an intensely pruritic eruption, usually affecting the web spaces of the fingers and volar aspect of the wrist. It can produce a generalised papular eruption or nodules if left untreated.

Schistosoma haematobium causes schistosomiasis.

Case 7

1   A   Spironolactone

This woman has facial hirsutism. Hirsutism is the abnormal growth of terminal hair in androgen-sensitive areas such as the moustache and beard regions. The causes of this are:

- Ovarian:
  PCOS
  ovarian hyperthecosis
  ovarian tumours
- Adrenal:
  congenital adrenal hyperplasia
  Cushing's disease
  adrenal tumours
- Hyperprolactinaemia
- Acromegaly
- Androgen therapy, eg anabolic steroids
- Idiopathic – can be racial variation.

Appropriate investigations include:

- Testosterone and sex hormone-binding globulin

- LH/FSH
- Androstenedione
- Dehydroepiandrosterone sulphate (DHEAS)
- Follicular phase 17-hydroxyprogesterone
- Prolactin
- Fasting glucose
- Ultrasound ovaries.

Treatment options are:

- Anti-androgen therapy:
    oral contraceptive
    cyproterone acetate
    spironolactone
    finasteride (5-α reductase inhibitor)
    dexamethasone (in CAH)
- Physical hair removal
- Waxing, shaving, electrolysis, laser.

Case 8

1   A   Fasting glucose

This is acanthosis nigricans. The characteristic clinical features are of hyperkeratosis, pigmentation, papillomatous elevations and a velvety texture to the skin. The sites most commonly involved are the axillae, neck, anal margin and groin flexures. It may also affect the submammary region, umbilicus and rarely the entire skin surface. A skin biopsy is not usually required as this is a typical appearance.

The causes of acanthosis nigricans are:

1   The metabolic syndrome – acanthosis is a marker of insulin resistance which visceral obesity may be a cause of. Hyperglycaemia (impaired fasting glucose, impaired glucose tolerance or frank type 2 diabetes mellitus), dysplipidaemia (elevated LDL and triglycerides and low HDL), hypertension, hyperuricaemia, elevated plasminogen activator, increased coronary artery disease and PCOS can all be features of the metabolic syndrome. Treatments that improve insulin sensitivity are weight loss and exercise, and hypoglycaemic agents. Insulin sensitisers, eg metformin and thiozoladinediones, are particularly attractive for treatment of the metabolic syndrome.
2   Hereditary benign acanthosis nigricans – this is determined by an irregular dominant gene. It is not associated with any endocrine abnormality.
3   Drug-induced – nicotinic acid, fusidic acid, stilbestrol and the oral contraceptive pill.

4   Malignant – usually in association with adenocarcinoma but also TCC bladder and SCC bronchus. Acanthosis developing after the age of 40 years is more suspicious of malignancy. Its occurrence in slender elderly people is highly suggestive of internal malignancy.

There is also condition called 'Pseudoacanthosis nigricans'. This is a benign and reversible complication of obesity. This is more commonly seen in skin types IV and V.

Case 9

1   **B**   Dermatomyositis

These are Gottron's papules, a pathognomonic sign in dermatomyositis. Other typical cutaneous manifestations of dermatomyositis include:

* Heliotropic (violaceous) inflammatory rash of the eyelids. There may also be periorbital oedema
* Erythema of the face, neck and upper trunk, which is often photosensitive
* Calcinosis
* Raynaud's phenomenon.

Extracutaneous features of dermatomyositis are:

* Muscle weakness – proximal myopathy, dysphagia, dysarthria
* Pulmonary fibrosis and pulmonary hypertension
* Myocarditis and myocardial fibrosis – conduction defects, cardiac failure
* Associated malignancy (in 10–50% cases) – lung, breast, ovarian, stomach, renal, testis.

Diagnosis is confirmed by:

* Skin biopsy
* Muscle biopsy
* Muscle MRI, which can replace the need for muscle biopsy and can identify patchy involvement (which can lead to a false-negative muscle biopsy).
* EMG
* ANA-positive in > 90% and anti-Jo-1 in 40%.

Other useful investigations include:

* ECG
* CXR.

This patient also requires chest CT and/or bronchoscopy.

The rash improves when an underlying malignancy is treated. Other therapies include:

- Systemic corticosteroids
- Hydroxychloroquine
- Methotrexate
- Intravenous immunoglobulin
- Sun protection.

Case 10

1   **C**   Pulsed intravenous methylprednisolone

This is a classic picture of pyoderma gangrenosum. Pyoderma gangrenosum is a destructive, necrotising, non-infective ulceration of the skin. It presents as an ulcer with an undermined, overhanging purple edge. There may be associated surrounding inflammation and necrosis.

Most cases of pyoderma gangrenosum are associated with an underlying disease process. These include:

- Gastrointestinal disease – ulcerative colitis, Crohn's disease, peptic ulcer disease
- Liver disease – chronic active hepatitis, primary biliary cirrhosis, sclerosing cholangitis
- Joint disease – rheumatoid arthritis, ankylosing spondylitis, osteoarthritis, polychondritis, Behçet's syndrome
- Blood disorders – leukaemias, myelomas, lymphomas
- Neoplasia – carcinoma of the colon, prostate, breast or bronchus and neuroendocrine tumours (carcinoids).

Pyoderma gangrenosum is often precipitated by trauma or surgery. Surgical debridement exacerbates the condition.

Treatment is with immunosuppressive therapy. Initially this involves high-dose steroids. Ciclosporin, azathioprine and methotrexate are often used. More recently, cytokine blocking agents (infliximab) have been used with success.

Case 11

1   **D**   Cutaneous leishmaniasis

This is a typical ulcer of cutaneous leishmaniasis. Leishmaniasis is transmitted by the sandfly. It can be cutaneous or visceral. Cutaneous leishmaniasis can be of 'Old World' or 'New World' types.

1   Old World cutaneous leishmaniasis
     Caused by *Leishmania major, L. tropica, L. aethiopica, L. infantum,*

and is endemic in the Eastern Mediterranean, Middle East, Southern Russia. There is some leishmaniasis in China, India and North Africa.

The incubation period is approximately 2 months.

It produces one or more lesions, usually on exposed sites. The sequence of disease is of a nodule which crusts, then forms an ulcer that heals slowly with scar formation.

2   New World mucocutaneous leishmaniasis

Caused by *L. braziliensis*, *L. mexicana*, and is endemic in South and Central America, especially in forest and jungle areas after the rainy season. It produces an ulcer, which may be verrucous ± lymphadenopathy. It can be aggressive and destroy cartilage.

40% of those affected develop mucosal lesions, usually in the nasal mucosa. It may present 2 years after infection.

Diagnosis:

- It is important to consider in travellers returning from endemic areas
- Smear of exudate from the sore: Giemsa or Wright's stain demonstrate the parasite
- Needle aspiration
- Culture
- Histology of an ulcer typically shows Leishman–Donovan bodies.

Treatment:

Sodium stibogluconate 20 mg/kg/day for 2–3 weeks.

Visceral leishmaniasis (kala-azar):

- *L. donovani* is usually the responsible agent
- Present with fever, fatigue, cough, diarrhoea, epistaxis, splenomegaly, hepatomegaly, lymphadenopathy and hyperpigmentation of the skin.

Case 12

1   **E**   Lichen planus

This is lichen planus. It characteristically causes small, flat-topped, violaceous papules over the wrists, ankles and genitalia. White lacy lines called 'Wickham's striae' are often seen within lesions. Oral involvement is common – usually white patches or plaques on the buccal mucosa, but sometimes erosive changes are seen. Nails typically have pitting, longitudinal ridging and distal splitting. Scalp involvement can be seen, with scarring alopecia which is then known as 'lichen planopilaris'.

Risk factors for lichen planus include:

- Chronic liver disease, especially hepatitis C
- Drugs – antimalarials, gold, penicillamine
- Colour film developers.

Treatment:

- Avoid predisposing factors
- Topical corticosteroids
- PUVA/UVB phototherapy
- Systemic immunosuppressants – including prednisolone, ciclosporin, and azathioprine – are required in some.

Scabies typically causes itchy papules too, but classically involves the finger web spaces. After 6 months' scabies infestation, one would expect to see scabetic nodules.

Secondary syphilis produces a non-itchy eruption over the upper extremities and trunk, with special predilection for the palms.
Eczema can produce itchy papules anywhere, but the Wickham's striae and underlying hepatitis C make lichen planus much more likely in this case.

Psoriasis is not itchy.

Case 13

1   **D**   Leprosy

The combination of a hypopigmented patch and ulnar nerve palsy is compatible with a diagnosis of leprosy, of borderline type.

Tuberculoid leprosy (TL) → borderline leprosy → lepromatous leprosy (LL)

Skin lesions:

- Sharply defined plaques
- Hypopigmented
- Anaesthetic skin lesions
- Symmetrical nodules or plaques
- May be hyperaesthetic.

Nerve lesions:

- Nerves near lesions may be enlarged
- Nerve trunk palsies
- Nerve palsies variable
- Distal symmetrical anaesthesia common.

Lepromin skin test:
Positive → negative → negative.

Acid-fast bacilli:
Rare (paucibacillary) → some → lots (multibacillary).

Leprosy is endemic in Asia, Africa, the Pacific Basin and Latin America. The average incubation period is 5 years. Transmission is probably via nasal droplets.

Treatment:

It needs to be more intensive in the multibacillary lepromatous type compared with the tuberculoid type
Dapsone + rifampicin + clofazimine for multibacillary LL
Dapsone + rifampicin for paucibacillary TL.

Complications:

1 Reversal reactions – these occur when treatment is initiated in patients with borderline disease. The disease shifts towards TL, existing lesions may become inflamed and tender, and new 'satellite' lesions may occur. Painful nerve trunk palsies may occur.
2 Erythema nodosum leprosum – this occurs in half of patients with LL. It usually develops within the first few years after treatment is initiated. It can affect any part of body and is self-limiting. There is associated fever, malaise, anorexia and anaemia.

Case 14

1 **C** Withdraw carbamazepine

This is toxic epidermal necrolysis. There is extensive full-thickness attachment of the epidermis. It is the most severe form of erythema multiforme. Typically the rash starts as poorly defined macules with darker centres. There is then sheet-like loss of the epidermis. Mucous membrane involvement is present in 95% of patients, with involvement of the oropharynx, eyes, genitalia and anus. High fever is usual.

Most cases are related to an adverse drug reaction. The commonest culprits are sulphonamides (eg co-trimoxazole), aromatic anticonvulsants (eg phenytoin, phenobarbital, carbamazepine), some NSAIDs (eg phenylbutazone, piroxicam) and allopurinol. The incidence is increased in patients with HIV infection. There is a high morbidity and mortality (30%) associated with this condition.

Complications:

• Fluid loss – replace with an extra 3–4 litres per day
• Infection – the main cause of death in these patients
• Impaired thermoregulation
• Increased energy expenditure.

Management:

- Withdraw any suspect drug
- Avoid skin trauma, including large intravascular lines
- Fluid replacement
- Needs ITU/burns unit bed
- Sterile handling of the patient
- Non-adherent skin dressings
- Nasogastric tube and high-protein diet
- Raise environmental temperature to 30–32 °C
- Ophthalmology examination daily.

Case 15

1   **B**   Rheumatoid arthritis

These pictures show two features – nail-fold infarcts and a symmetrical polyarthropathy with swelling of the MCP joints.

Nail-fold infarcts are seen in association with small-vessel vasculitis. They are characteristically seen in rheumatoid arthritis, SLE, scleroderma and dermatomyositis.

Only 30% of patients with rheumatoid arthritis are ANA-positive (cf SLE, 85%).

Chapter Two   Answers

ENDOCRINOLOGY AND METABOLISM

Case 1

1   E   Familial dysbetalipoproteinaemia

There is a combined hyperlipidaemia with striate palmar xanthomas. Palmar xanthomata are almost diagnostic of familial dysbetalipoproteinaemia, (synonyms are broad-beta disease, remnant removal disease or type III hyperlipidaemia (Fredrickson/WHO classification)). Tuberoeruptive xanthomas also occur and may coalesce to form tuberous xanthomas. Untreated, there is a marked increased incidence of coronary heart disease and peripheral vascular disease. It is rare; treatment is with diet, fibrates or statins. In the absence of palmar xanthomas it cannot be distinguished from familial combined hyperlipidaemia (type IIb) or lipoprotein lipase deficiency (type V or I hyperlipidaemia) on simple lipid measurement alone. Most (90%) of the patients are homozygous for apolipoprotein E ε2. DNA testing for this is troublesome because it may identify the presence of ε4 which is linked with early-onset Alzheimer's disease; this information should not be openly available in the patient's notes without their consent. Plasma can also be examined by ultracentrifugation for the presence of β-VLDL (hence broad-beta), typical of familial dysbetalipoproteinaemia. About 1% of the population have the ε2/ε2 phenotype; they have cholesterol- enriched VLDL and low LDL, but do not have type III dysbetalipoproteinaemia, whose expression requires the co-existence of a further abnormality affecting lipid metabolism. Examples of this are hypothyroidism and obesity. Note that the total cholesterol is not made up of LDL and this suggests elevated IDL which is characteristic of dysbetalipoproteinaemia. The disorder responds to weight reduction, fibrates and statins. The high triglycerides confer an elevated risk of pancreatitis.

Patients with familial mixed hyperlipidaemia have increased VLDL (triglycerides) and LDL and typically low HDL; they are prone to coronary artery disease, stroke and peripheral vascular disease. Treatment is with diet and weight loss, statins, nicotinic acid and fibrates. The hyperlipidaemia of diabetes most closely resembles this.

Patients with familial hypercholesterolaemia have increased LDL due to a defect in the LDL receptor inherited in an autosomal dominant manner. Heterozygosity is present in the UK in ~1:450 people; their LDL-receptor activity is reduced by ~50%. The commonest presentation, unless picked up by screening, is early-onset ischaemic heart disease. Tendon and planar xanthomas occur. It responds to diet, statins, ezetimibe, bile-acid binding resins, nicotinic acid and fibrates.

Patients with familial hypertriglyceridaemia have elevated chylomicrons and VLDL, with very elevated triglycerides in the serum – stored plasma has a milky, lipaemic top (due to chylomicrons). Eruptive xanthomas on the extensor surfaces and lipaemia retinalis occur. Pancreatitis occurs but an increased risk of ischaemic heart disease is debated. Pseudohyponatraemia can occur. It responds to a very low fat diet, fibrates, omega-3 fatty acids and nicotinic acid.

Case 2

1   **C**   Referral to an ophthalmic surgeon

There is a 1.5–2-cm soft-tissue-density retro-orbital mass arising from within the right orbit, from either the greater wing of the sphenoid, the fronto or the zygomatic bones. The orbit itself is proptosed. An ophthalmic surgeon should be consulted in case the lesion is malignant or there are compressive problems; benign retro-orbital tumours can grow very slowly and just be kept under observation. Note that the medial rectus muscles are of normal size – these are characteristically involved in Graves' ophthalmopathy.

The thyroid scan shows several signal voids within the gland, suggesting a multinodular gland. If this is in keeping with the exam findings, then she could be followed up clinically or with ultrasound. The use of fine-needle aspiration cytology depends on local practice.

There is little evidence that suppressive doses of thyroxine help suppress the growth of goitres. Lack of evidence of benefit does not equate to evidence of no benefit – many thyroidologists therefore still use suppressive thyroxine. However, there is evidence that patients with a suppressed TSH have adverse morbidity and mortality.

Case 3

1   **C**   Cranial diabetes insipidus

Considering the problem of polyuria, the following diagnoses need to be considered:

- Diabetes mellitus
- Diabetes insipidus (DI):
       cranial
       nephrogenic
- Primary polydipsia (PP)
- Polyuric phase of renal failure.

Diabetes mellitus is excluded by the normal fasting glucose, absence of glucose on urinalysis and lack of weight loss. The + ketones is normal for a fasting urine. Polyuria is present as the 24-hour urine output is over 2.5 L. There are no clinical features here to distinguish between the remaining causes. Clues however could be:

- Psychosis – primary polydipsia
- Evidence of pituitary or hypothalamic disease – cranial DI.

There is no hypokalaemia or hypercalcaemia, renal failure or evidence of pituitary or hypothalamic disease. The basal osmolalities show a moderately concentrated plasma (this mild dehydration, together with a high sodium and albumin tends to favour DI; in PP one often sees an plasma osmolality below 280 mosmol/kg due to a degree of overhydration) with a low urine osmolality (the latter is unhelpful for distinguishing between mild DI and PP). One would imagine from first principles that in PP the urine would concentrate if the plasma became concentrated. However, with any cause of chronic polyuria there is a solute washout from the renal medulla which reduces renal concentrating ability, hence the low urine osmolality is unhelpful.

A water deprivation test is the usual investigation to do at this stage. Here the urine osmolality fails to rise appropriately and urine volume remains high despite the rising plasma osmolality. Once the plasma osmolality has risen above 295 mosmol/kg, the patient has been adequately water-deprived and DDAVP is given. Now urine concentrates normally. This is diagnostic of cranial DI.

In nephrogenic DI the urine would fail to concentrate after DDAVP. In PP one might not see the plasma concentrate to over 295 mosmol/kg, and the urine to plasma osmolality ratio may remain less than 2.0. If so, either a prolonged water deprivation test (Miller and Moses) or AVP measurement during hypertonic saline infusion could be performed.

Case 4

1   **E**   Primary hyperparathyroidism (PHP)

The baseline biochemistry shows hypercalcaemia, the corrected calcium is 3.0 mmol/L (albumin is 41 g/L), the phosphate is low and there is a normal anion gap metabolic acidosis. The 24-hour calcium is elevated, highly suggestive of PHP. PTH increases serum calcium by mobilising it from bone and increasing proximal tubular resorption and increases both phosphate and bicarbonate excretion by preventing their resorption in the proximal tubule.

The PTH is not suppressed, suggesting one of three diagnoses:

- Primary hyperparathyroidism (PHP)

- Tertiary hyperparathyroidism (THP)
- Familial hypercalcaemic hypocalciuria (FHH).

There is no cause for THP – the renal function is normal and vitamin D deficiency, severe enough to cause THP, is unlikely with the normal ALP (but **possible** with the early-onset osteoporosis), and malabsorption is not suggested.

FHH is not present as the 24-hour urinary calcium is far too high at 9.165 mmol/day. It should not be necessary to calculate the calcium/creatinine clearance ratio with the 24-hour calcium excretion, but it is > 0.01, against the diagnosis of FHH.

urine [Ca^{2+}] × plasma [creatinine] / urine [Ca^{2+}] × plasma [creatinine]

This formula is only valid if both calcium and creatinine are measured on the same 24-hour urine. PHP has its highest incidence in the fourth to sixth decades when it is twice as common in women; in all other age groups the incidence is equal. In the UK hospital population, where routine measurement of serum calcium is common, an incidence of at least 1% is revealed. Most (99%) have benign tumours (85% adenomas and 15% multiple abnormal glands) and 1% have carcinoma. PHP can be part of familial multiple endocrine neoplasia syndromes and this should be considered if there is a family history of hypercalcaemia or other endocrine neoplasia or when PHP occurs in the young. The depression, Colles' fracture at age 51 and the suggestion of diabetes insipidus all push one towards definitive management – surgical parathyroidectomy.

FHH is transmitted in an autosomal dominant fashion and is due (in most) to a mutation in the calcium-sensing-receptor gene. Consider if there is a history of unsuccessful neck or parathyroid surgery. It is best diagnosed by a calcium/creatinine clearance ratio < 0.01.

In this case the hypertension is a red herring. One might consider MEN 2A but there is nothing to suggest a phaeochromocytoma; essential hypertension is common. If it were MEN 2A, medullary carcinoma of the thyroid usually (but not exclusively) would have occurred by now.

Case 5

1   **B**   Anterior pituitary function

In the presence of hypoglycaemia there is an inadequate serum cortisol. Therefore one can confidently say that hypoadrenalism exists. A short tetracosactrin test will give no more useful information – the patient has essentially had an insulin tolerance test.

The next question is whether it is primary or secondary hypoadrenalism.

Primary adrenal failure would cause mineralocorticoid and glucocorticoid deficiency. The clinical information in this scenario does not point to mineralocorticoid deficiency as the volume status of the patient is normal, the JVP is 4 cm and there is no postural drop; the image shows an absence of secondary sexual hair – suggesting hypogonadism; the electrolytes are, at best, not suggestive of mineralocorticoid deficiency or, at worst, unhelpful. The image does not show pigmentation which would favour Addison's disease. All this points to pituitary or hypothalamic disease rather than to primary adrenal disease – measuring ACTH is mandatory if one suspects Addison's but is not mandatory here. The stress of a general anaesthetic has precipitated a crisis. Due to glucocorticoid deficiency he will have inadequate liver glycogen stores, especially after a fast for a general anaesthetic, hence severe hypoglycaemia has occurred; one may think the blood pressure is a little low for the clinical scenario too.

Anterior pituitary function tests should therefore be performed and the visual fields should be assessed with some urgency in case there is a lesion compressing the optic chiasm – which can go unnoticed.

The possibility of an insulinoma ought to be considered, but the patient has an alternative cause for hypoglycaemia and also has urinary ketones. These indicate a low prevailing burden of insulin in the body during the fast and suggest that insulin, an insulin-like peptide (eg pro-IGF-II from a sarcoma) or sulphonylureas are not to blame.

Case 6

1   **B**   Distal renal tubular acidosis – RTA (type 1)

The clinical details are of an arrhythmia in a well young lady who has some aches and pains and a proximal myopathy. The investigations show a normal anion gap metabolic acidosis with marked hypokalaemia.

The causes of a normal anion gap metabolic acidosis include:

- Distal renal tubular acidosis (type 1) – hypokalaemic
- Distal renal tubular acidosis (type 4) – hyperkalaemic:
    Addison's disease
    mineralocorticoid resistance
    hyporeninaemia:
        autonomic failure (Shy–Drager)
        diabetes mellitus
- Proximal renal tubular acidosis (type 2).

The abdominal X-ray shows nephrocalcinosis, the causes of which are summarised in the list at the top of the next page.

- Mainly medullary (the usual location ~95%):
  primary hyperparathyroidism ⎫
  distal RTA (type 1) ⎬ 60% of cases
  ⎭
  idiopathic hypercalciuria
  hypervitaminosis D
  milk alkali syndrome
  primary hyperoxaluria
  sarcoidosis
  chronic berylliosis
  thyrotoxicosis
  sulphonamide injury
- Mainly cortical (< 5%):
  chronic glomerulonephritis
  renal cortical necrosis with recovery ('tram-line' calcification)
- Medullary cystic disease: to some authorities, this is not considered to be a cause of nephrocalcinosis. It causes calcification at the tips of the papillae, not in the medulla. There is cystic dilatation of the collecting ducts with calcification within these.

Hypokalaemia (see p. 160) is responsible for the myopathy and the arrhythmia. Arrhythmias associated with hypokalaemia include:

- Atrial tachycardia with block
- Atrioventricular dissociation (hence cannon waves in the JVP)
- Ventricular tachycardia or fibrillation.

The ECG shows prominent U waves and small T waves (that can often be lost within the U wave); this can give the false appearance of a prolonged QT interval.

Hypokalaemia also reduces gut motility and can cause a frank ileus. However in ileus there is no pain and bowel sounds are absent, so the abdominal pain is possibly due to calcium nephrolithiasis.

The only unifying diagnosis is distal RTA (type 1).

The causes of distal RTA (type 1) are as follows:

- Autoimmune disease:
  Sjögren's syndrome
  primary biliary cirrhosis and other autoimmune liver disease
  SLE
  cryoglobulinaemia
- Associated with nephrocalcinosis:
  primary hyperparathyroidism
  vitamin D toxicity
- Tubulointerstitial nephropathy:
  chronic pyelonephritis

chronic obstruction
renal transplantation
- Inherited:
autosomal dominant or, rarely autosomal recessive
sickle cell anaemia
medullary sponge kidney
- Drug-related:
analgesic nephropathy
amphotericin B.

In this case the other features to note are a mild renal impairment consistent with volume contraction, which exacerbates the secondary hyperaldosteronism. There is perhaps a clue to the aetiology in this youngish lady with a high ALP – primary biliary cirrhosis – or this could represent the osteomalacia that frequently complicates the acidosis. The autosomal dominant form can present in adulthood but more normally it presents in childhood with failure to thrive.

In proximal RTA (type 2) nephrocalcinosis is almost never present; there are usually multiple defects of tubular function and the urine pH can become normal with a severe acidosis.

Case 7

1   C   MRI pituitary

The history is absolutely classic for pituitary apoplexy. The preceding headache may allude to the growth of a pituitary tumour, and the fatigue and weight loss may allude to thyrotrophic and corticotrophic hormone failure respectively. There is no clue to the state of the gonadotrophic hormones because of the combined pill. The diplopia and VIth nerve palsy are due to compression within the cavernous sinus on the left; the cavernous sinuses lie just lateral to the pituitary fossa and through it travel cranial nerves III, IV, Va, Vb and VI – any or all can be affected as can the optic chiasm. The fields must therefore be checked forthwith as compression of the chiasm changes the tempo of the case and injects extreme urgency. If there is any visual loss, then operative decompression ought to occur within the first week.

There is no evidence to suggest SIADH as the patient is volume-deplete, tachycardic with a low BP, and becomes dizzy on standing. The osmolalities are confusing if one has not made the correct assessment of volume status.

A sensible clinician may send the CSF to virology but it will not give you the diagnosis. Similarly, cortisol should be measured as we are concerned about the pituitary, but ACTH will add nothing. Even cortisol on its own would not be the correct answer. Note the CSF glucose is low and if it is 70% of the plasma, then there is a low plasma glucose too.

Case 8

1   C   Langerhans' cell histiocytosis (LCH)

The calculated serum osmolality, (2 × [Na + K] + (glucose + urea) is 304 mosmol/kg, yet the urine is dilute, suggesting a failure of urinary concentrating ability. The patient is being investigated for diabetes, but has not lost any weight; one can assume that polyuria and/or polydipsia raised the possibility of diabetes – the plasma glucose is normal – therefore diabetes insipidus is almost certainly present.

Specific gravity	Osmolality (mosmol/kg)
1.002	100
1.010	285
1.020	750
1.030	1200
1.035	1400

There are lucencies on the skull vault, the cause which may be:

- LCH
- Metastases
- Hyperparathyroidism
- Burr hole
- Neurofibroma
- Multiple myeloma
- Paget's disease
- Haemangioma
- Infective, eg tuberculosis.

The patient also has a rash, unsuccessfully treated as seborrhoeic eczema. A rash is the most frequent feature of LCH, but it is often overlooked. This, together with skull lucencies and diabetes insipidus, makes Langerhans' cell histiocytosis the only correct answer. A tissue biopsy should ideally be performed to confirm this. Full anterior pituitary function tests should be performed. The disease can remit spontaneously and if it is not causing any trouble, can be observed.

The lucencies were present in childhood, making metastases unlikely; the patient is too young for myeloma. It is not the pepper-pot skull of hyperparathyroidism. There are no other features in the case to suggest neurofibromatosis.

Case 9

1   **A**   Primary aldosteronism – bilateral adrenal hyperplasia

There is hypertension and evidence of mineralocorticoid (MC) excess – an alkalosis with the potassium in the lower part of the normal range. Up to 40% of patients with surgically confirmed primary aldosteronism have normal serum potassium; the alkalosis reflects intracellular potassium depletion.

The next step in the investigation is to look at the plasma renin. Suppression is compatible with primary aldosteronism; if it is not suppressed, primary aldosteronism is very unlikely. To increase the predictive value of this test, it is best performed on a diet with at least 100 mmol sodium per day, though this is a matter of diagnostic finesse rather than a critical fact for MRCP purposes.

One would normally expect to see that the aldosterone is elevated as the most likely diagnosis is primary aldosteronism (Conn's syndrome). Conn's syndrome is an acceptable term for primary aldosteronism caused by either unilateral adenoma or bilateral adrenal hyperplasia.

Considering mineralocorticoid hypertension more formally, the causes are as follows:

- Normal MC receptor, normal ligand:
    primary aldosteronism
    glucocorticoid-remediable hyperaldosteronism (GRA)
- Normal receptor, abnormal ligand:
    apparent MC excess (AME):
        11β-hydroxysteroid dehydrogenase (HSD) deficiency
        11β-HSD inactivation (glycyrrhetinic acid – liquorice, carbenoxolone)
    deoxycorticosterone (DOC) excess:
        adrenal tumour – DOComa
        congenital adrenal hyperplasia:
            11-hydroxylase deficiency
            17-hydroxylase deficiency
- Constitutive activation of receptor
    progesterone- (P_2)- induced hypertension (autosomal dominant inheritance)
- Increased post-receptor activation:
    Liddle's syndrome.

In our case the aldosterone is raised, confirming primary aldosteronism.

The imaging shows normal adrenals, making bilateral adrenal hyperplasia likely. There is a case to be made for going on to do postural renin aldosterone studies and possibly a venous catheter for aldosterone. A therapeutic mistake can be made by performing a unilateral adrenalectomy on a patient with bilateral disease. Remember that incidental adrenal masses are common.

Bartter's syndrome does not cause hypertension. In Liddle's syndrome the aldosterone is low. Phaeochromocytomas are often associated with a postural drop and the urine catecholamines are typically raised.

Case 10

1   E   The statin should be discontinued

One would consider a rise in the transaminases of over three times the upper limit of normal as a reason to discontinue the statin; otherwise, they ought not to be discontinued. Increasing evidence shows that statins are safe to initiate early after myocardial infarction (MI), and clinical practice in the UK would be not to stop.

The management of MI in diabetes (of whatever type) is along standard lines for non-diabetics. Retinopathy does not preclude thrombolysis. Patients with diabetes have a worse prognosis after MI than non-diabetics but have a greater benefit from thrombolysis and should always receive thrombolysis (or primary angioplasty) whatever the stage of retinopathy.[1]

The absolute benefit of ACE inhibitors post-infarct is clear from several trials and neither the renal impairment nor proteinuria preclude their use. The presence of a third heart sound, even in the absence of pulmonary oedema, is a clear indication of left ventricular dysfunction, which one would expect in anterior infarction.

Beta-blockers are not contraindicated after MI in diabetes and they reduce mortality, sudden cardiac death and re-infarction after MI. The loss of hypoglycaemic awareness is inconsequential. Intravenous β-blockade is more difficult, the evidence is contradictory but, on balance, they are probably beneficial, although the effect may be smaller than previously thought.[2] In the presence of hypertension that precludes thrombolysis, β-blockers will lower the BP and allow thrombolysis to be given. The matter in this question is easier as the systolic pressure precludes intravenous β-blockade.

[1] Aiello LP, Cahill MT, Wong JS. 2001. Systemic considerations in the management of diabetic retinopathy. *American Journal of Ophthalmology*, 132, 760–776.
[2] Borrello F, Beahan M, Klein L, Gheorghiade M. 2003. Reappraisal of beta-blocker therapy in the acute and chronic post-myocardial infarction period. *Review of Cardiovascular Medicine*, 4(suppl 3): S13–S24.

Case 11

1   C   Chronic pancreatitis

The image shows pancreatic calcification across the abdomen at the level of the first lumbar vertebra, which is almost diagnostic of chronic pancreatitis. Intermittent, boring pain through to the back is characteristic and the suggestion that he stopped drinking because of abdominal pain is evidence of the aetiology. There is a mild anaemia and a faint macrocytosis – this could be due to B_{12} deficiency, which is occasionally found in chronic pancreatitis. The capillary glucose is 7.9 mmol/L and although we do not know whether the patient had eaten recently, this must make one think of either diabetes mellitus or impaired glucose tolerance – the appropriate diagnostic samples must be taken. A mild obstructive jaundice is a frequent finding; malabsorption of fat-soluble vitamins is common, but clinical manifestations such as osteomalacia are rare.

Carcinoma of the head of the pancreas is a possibility but the pain is more relentless, weight loss more of a feature, and the jaundice occurs earlier in carcinoma; pancreatic calcification is less of a feature – but chronic pancreatitis can develop in the pancreas proximal to an obstructing carcinoma. Pancreatic carcinoma has a mean age of onset of 55 years, and the duration of symptoms is less than 6 months in half of patients; the average duration of symptoms before death is between 4 and 10 months.

There is nothing to suggest metastases or tuberculous adrenal disease.

Case 12

1   D   McArdle's disease

This patient's history goes back to childhood and he is now an underweight adult with proximal wasting and normal reflexes (MRCP-speak for a myopathy).

The causes of myopathy are:

- Endocrine:
    hypocalcaemia
    hypokalaemia
    hypomagnesaemia
    hypo- or hyperthyroidism
    Cushing's syndrome
    glycogen storage disorders
    lipid storage diseases
    mitochondrial diseases

periodic paralyses
- Inflammatory:
  polymyositis
  dermatomyositis
- Toxic:
  corticosteroids
  statins
  colchicine
  amiodarone
  alcohol
  penicillamine
  halothane – malignant hyperpyrexia
  vincristine
  chloroquine.

There is blood in the dipstick urinalysis but no cells or casts are seen on microscopy, suggesting myoglobinuria. This occurs in muscle injury or damage, as in:

- Trauma/compression
- Exercise
- Burns and electric shocks
- Viral myositis
- Sepsis – gas gangrene, tetanus, Legionnaires', shigellosis
- Malignant hyperpyrexia
- Coma
- Seizures
- Metabolic myopathies:
  hypokalaemia
  glycogen storage disorders
  mitochondrial diseases
  lipid storage disorders
  defects of carbohydrate metabolism
- Drugs/toxins – AZT, statins, ethylene glycol, isopropyl alcohol, phencyclidine
- Snake bites.

The metabolic myopathies present with exercise intolerance and cramps and myoglobinuria. Cramps and muscle discomfort may occur after brief exercise (as in this case) or prolonged activity. Glycogen is the main source of energy during brief exercise, while fatty acids are more important in prolonged exercise. These cramps occurring early favour glycogen storage disease.

There are several glycogen storage diseases. Pompé's usually presents in children but can rarely present in an adult with a limb-girdle dystrophic picture. McArdle's (due to muscle phosphorylase deficiency), presenting with exertional cramps early during exercise, is associated with elevations of LDH, creatine kinase and myoglobinuria. Patients have a normal lifespan and there is no association with hepatomegaly.

There is no hypothalamo-pituitary-adrenal axis pathology (the cortisol of 170 nmol/L does not have a sampling time).

Case 13

1   C   Impaired glucose tolerance

This question requires a practical knowledge of the diagnostic criteria for normality, impaired fasting glucose (IFG), impaired glucose tolerance (IGF), and diabetes mellitus (DM). While these are complex, they must be simplified to be practically useful. They are important as we are habitually faced with interpreting glucose levels.

One must identify normality and identify when normality is not present. Furthermore one must identify who to investigate more intensively (or suggest that the GP investigates further) with surveillance, repeat testing or, rarely, an oral glucose tolerance test (OGTT).

The importance of diagnosing diabetes mellitus is apparent. However, the importance of diagnosing both impaired fasting glucose and impaired glucose tolerance is often overlooked. IFG and IGT identify patients who are at increased risk of developing diabetes; some 5% per year, or 30% at 10 years. They also identify patients who are at increased risk of developing macrovascular disease. Prospective data is sparse but it seems that the risk of progression to DM and macrovascular disease is greater with IGT than with IFG. Their other macrovascular risk factors must be addressed.

There is no substitute for looking at the full WHO guidelines on the diagnosis of diabetes but they are cumbersome.[1] The following points **must** be taken with the proviso that samples must be repeated in asymptomatic individuals; hyperglycaemia must be interpreted with extreme caution in those with acute infective, traumatic, circulatory or other stress as it may be transitory.

It is helpful to remember that, **broadly speaking**:
On fasting venous plasma samples:

$\leqslant$6.0 mmol/L suggests normality;
$\geqslant$7.0 mmol/L suggests diabetes;
in-between is IFG.

After a 75 g glucose load:
$\geqslant$11.1 mmol/L suggests diabetes;

< 7.8 suggests normality;
in-between is IGT.

A random value of:
5.5 mmol/L strongly suggests normality;
≥ 11.1 mmol/L suggests DM.

[1] http://www.diabetes.org.uk/infocentre/carcrec/newdiagnotic.htm

Case 14

1   D   Hydrocortisone 100 mg intravenously stat and 20 mg orally tds

The clinical scenario is hyponatraemia. There is a major clue to a
possible aetiology in that she takes inhalers for mild COPD, possibly
suggesting steroids.

The first part of establishing the aetiology is establishing the volume
status of the patient. The following table outlines the possible causes
based on the volume.

Hypovolaemic	Euvolaemic	Hypervolaemic
Diuretics	SIADH	Heart failure
Type 4 RTA: • Diabetes mellitus • Mineralocorticoid deficiency, eg Addison's disease or isolated aldosterone deficiency • Mineralocorticoid resistance, eg spironolactone	Glucocorticoid deficiency Hypothyroidism Sick cell concept Inappropriate intravenous fluids, eg dextrose	Renal: • Acute and chronic renal failure • Nephrotic syndrome Liver cirrhosis Inappropriate intravenous fluids
Salt-wasting nephropathy: • Post-obstruction • Tubulointerstitial nephropathy • Pyelonephritis		
Cerebral salt wasting		
Severe osmotic diuresis		
Other loss • Gut eg vomiting, diarrhoea • Excess sweating • Burns		

The commonest causes in hospital are hypovolaemia, due to either diuretics or vomiting, and SIADH. A lot is made of the biochemistry of SIADH and the urine and plasma osmolalities, but these tests can be identical in hypovolaemia and SIADH. Remember that the response of the body to hypovolaemia is to have an appropriate secretion of ADH.

This case however is clinically euvolaemic; there is no postural rise in pulse or fall in BP and the JVP is normal. The former two are the best tests for hypovolaemia; the JVP is under the influence of venous tone as well as volume. Beware of thinking of dehydration and hypovolaemia as synonymous; this is an extremely common and ill-thought-out practice, which leads to confusion.

As the patient is euvolaemic, we now consider the causes of euvolaemic hyponatraemia. She has an inappropriate morning cortisol, especially as she is post-operative; taken in the context of the rather low blood pressure must make one consider the hypothalamo-pituitary-adrenal axis more closely. She has been on inhalers and so is likely to have a degree of adrenal suppression, causing hyponatraemia. This is quite common and often ignored, but glucocorticoids are important stress hormones and she needs to be rendered eucortisolaemic. Glucocorticoid deficiency contributes to hypotension in deficiency states by decreasing vascular responsiveness to angiotensin II, norepinephrine and other vasoconstrictive hormones, reducing the synthesis of renin substrate, and increasing production and effects of prostacyclin and other vasodilatory hormones. However they are protected against adrenal crises by an intact zona glomerulosa producing aldosterone, which is in direct contrast to primary adrenal failure, when hypovolaemia and circulatory collapse can occur. (See also p. 173)

There are several ways to replace glucocorticoids, including parenterally, but this lady can swallow, her symptoms and biochemical disturbance are mild; 100 mg intravenously stat with a tablet at the same time is reasonable, but full parenteral replacement may be necessary.

Fluid restriction is often used in these circumstances but is not the correct thing to do. SIADH is a diagnosis of exclusion and hypoadrenalism and hypothyroidism cannot be present to make this diagnosis.

Intravenous fluid may be necessary but it is not the best answer.

Diabetes insipidus would cause hypernatraemia.

Case 15

1 **C** Subacute thyroiditis

2 **D** Radioactive iodine uptake scan

The story is typical of a subacute (de Quervain's) thyroiditis with acute onset of pain, sore throat and some dysphagia. There is a mild fever (it can be up to 40 °C and this must make one think of suppurative thyroiditis) and a firm goitre, which is tender in 75% of cases. The clinical findings are suggestive of thyrotoxicosis and the eyes show lid retraction, the sclera visible **above** the superior limbus of the cornea: this is a sign of sympathetic overactivity, together with the tremor and tachycardia. In this clinical scenario one will expect the TSH to be suppressed and the free thyroid hormone levels might be high. Thyroglobulin is elevated but it is not diagnostic. The ESR being elevated and the mild leucocytosis support the diagnosis, the former being a very helpful finding. The characteristic finding is decreased radioiodine uptake. The disease is thought to occur secondary to a viral inflammation of the gland where the entire preformed hormone is spilled out, causing hyperthyroidism; there then classically follows a period of euthyroidism, then hypothyroidism and subsequent recovery. Each period **classically** lasts 2 months.

Haemorrhage into a cyst is an even more abrupt presentation and a fluctuant swelling may be found. Ultrasound may help diagnose this condition; FNA can relieve the pressure and show diagnostic blood.

Graves' might be a possibility, but the history is too short, the goitre is tender and there is no exophthalmos (where the sclera is visible **below** the inferior limbus of the cornea, although this is only present in 33% of patients). The cardinal features of Graves' disease are ophthalmopathy (exophthalmos), dermopathy (pre-tibial myxoedema), acropachy and, some authors say, a diffuse, smooth goitre with a bruit. Note that biochemical thyroid dysfunction is not a necessary feature of Graves' disease. The diagnosis is often clinical and supported by the presence of thyroid peroxidase/microsomal or antithyroglobulin antibodies (thyroid-stimulating autoantibodies are not routinely assayed).

Riedel's thyroiditis is a very rare condition, most common between 30 and 60 years and twice as common in males. It causes a hard woody infiltration of the thyroid and surrounding tissues. There may be associated mediastinal or retroperitoneal fibrosis and sclerosing cholangitis.

Case 16

1   **D**   Adrenal cortex and 21-hydroxylase autoantibodies

The history is absolutely classic for adrenal hypofunction. The commonest symptom of chronic cortisol insufficiency is weight loss, often associated with episodes of vomiting and diarrhoea. Non-specific, colicky abdominal pain can occur over many months as attacks come and go; between attacks, lassitude and lack of energy are common complaints. Acute attacks can often lead to admission with shock, hypotension and hyponatraemia – addisonian crisis. The cortisol is low (at the low end of the normal range) in the morning but there is nothing to suggest either primary or secondary failure in the history. Secondary dysfunction is most commonly due to pharmacological steroid therapy. If there is evidence of other pituitary dysfunction it is a pointer towards secondary failure – the most common dysfunction is reproductive failure. If there is pigmentation it suggests primary dysfunction – it is not always present and remember that vitiligo is an association of Addison's.

In this case we have additional information – the ACTH is extremely elevated (normal range < 18 pmol/L). This clinches the diagnosis of primary adrenal failure – Addison's disease. There is no diagnostic advantage whatsoever in doing a tetracosactrin test in this patient.

To make it clear what the diagnosis is, let us imagine the cortisol and ACTH were T_4 and TSH. We would have a T_4 right at the lower end of the normal range, and a TSH some ten times elevated, such as:

T_4 11.1 pmol/L
TSH   40.3 mU/L

This must make one diagnose primary thyroid failure. It is no different with a cortisol and an ACTH, so one diagnoses primary adrenal failure and must now proceed to consider the aetiology. In the west this is autoimmune in up to 68–94% of cases and an antibody test is therefore the next step.

ACTH is a difficult hormone to assay and that leads to the short tetracosactrin test being used to try to exclude adrenal failure. This is not an altogether unreasonable clinical/laboratory practice but it can potentially miss secondary adrenal failure, particularly if it is of short duration as the adrenal cortical reserve to ACTH may still allow a normal test.

If the short tetracosactrin test indicates adrenal failure, a long test can be performed to elucidate whether it is primary or secondary. In secondary failure the adrenals can be stimulated at 24 hours. This test has largely been superseded by the increasing availability of ACTH assays.

The insulin tolerance test is the gold standard test for the whole hypothalamo-pituitary-adrenal axis (ACTH reserve) and growth hormone reserve.

Very-long-chain fatty acids can be assayed if one suspects X-linked adrenoleukodystrophy. This is X-linked recessive and consequently is vanishingly rare in females. In a male one should have a high clinical suspicion for adrenoleukodystrophy as it is frequently missed; it is a cause of primary adrenal failure in 20–35% of male cases in some series. There are obvious genetic counselling issues.

Tuberculous adrenalitis should be considered if antibodies are negative or present in low titres and a genetic syndrome is not likely/found. The definitive test is adrenal imaging to look for enlargement ± calcification.

Case 17

1   **D**   Change the nocturnal Insulatard® to insulin glargine

This answer should be taken in conjunction with the NICE guidelines for management of T1DM (adults)[1], and practical diabetes experience is useful. Insulin glargine – one of the long-acting analogues – has a much smoother time-course of action, with less of a peak in the middle of the night. It also lasts for a full 24 hours and thus can provide adequate control outside of mealtimes, particularly where analogues are used. NICE recommends glargine as the long-acting insulin where either lispro or aspart (the rapid-acting analogues) are used for pre-meal control; also use glargine when nocturnal hypoglycaemia is a problem or morning hyperglycaemia leads to poor control throughout the day.

There is no place for adding in metformin – the routine use of oral hypoglycaemics in T1DM is to be avoided. One can estimate a patient's sensitivity quickly with the knowledge that a sensitive individual will need about 0.5–0.6 U/kg of insulin; this lady therefore ought to be on about 42 units of insulin a day. In fact she is taking about that or perhaps a little more. One of the reasons she may have a degree of insulin resistance is the counter-regulatory hormones being released at night when she has hypos. Where there is clear evidence of insulin resistance in type 1 diabetes, as in abdominal obesity, metformin can be a useful adjunct. Examining the regime as a whole, one would expect about 30–50% of the total insulin to come from the basal component and the rest to be divided between the meals, depending on prevailing calories and exercise.

There is no evidence of either coeliac or Addison's – that 9-am cortisol would not explain hypoglycaemia. If Addison's were considered, the correct test to perform would be an ACTH, although most centres would actually do a short tetracosactrin test first as ACTH is still not a routine assay in the UK.

[1] http://www.nice.org.uk/pdf/CG015adultsquickrefguide.pdf

Case 18

1   **E**   Paget's disease

There is asymmetry of the femurs. There is expansion of the cortex and medulla and a coarse trabecular pattern within the cancellous bone right up to the femoral neck. The asymmetry, increased width of the bone and the trabeculation all point to Paget's.

There are three distinct appearances of the bones in Paget's on X-ray, all of which may be present within the same bone:

- Predominantly lytic disease, eg osteoporosis circumscripta in the skull
- Diffuse increase in density with bone enlargement
- New bone growth from the cortex into the medulla with enlargement and trabeculation of the bone.

The pelvis is the commonest site of Paget's disease. The distribution of the lesions within a bone is variable, sometimes the distal end, sometimes the proximal end and sometimes the whole bone is involved. The skull, long bones and spine are also commonly affected. It occurs in 10% of those over 80 and is twice as common in men than in women.

Hyperparathyroidism only shows radiological evidence in 10% of cases. Subperiosteal bone resorption can be seen at the radial side of the phalanx of the middle fingers, the lateral ends of the clavicles, medial aspect of the proximal tibia, pubic symphysis and the medial aspect of the neck of the femur. Brown tumours – focal lytic lesions, indicating local destruction due to intense osteoclastic activity, are most commonly seen in the mandible, pelvis, femora and ribs. The terminal tufts of the phalanges may be resorbed. In the skull, pepper-pot skull may be seen.

Osteomalacia causes a generalised loss of bone density. The main radiological features are stress fractures or pseudofractures (Looser's zones).

Acromegaly is a systemic disease and does not cause asymmetrical disease like this.

Metastatic prostatic carcinoma classically causes sclerotic bone lesions which are typically discrete but which can coalesce to become more confluent lesions.

Case 19

1   C   Charcot's foot

2   E   Immobilisation and total-contact cast

The history is suggestive of a neuropathic joint in that there is evidence of inflammation but it is not painful. The bones of the mid-foot (tarsals) are involved. There is bone and joint destruction and some bone fragmentation. This is Charcot's destructive arthropathy. The next commonest site in the foot is the first and second tarsometatarsal joints.

The first problem is differentiating this from osteomyelitis. This, however, is less likely if there is no ulceration and osteomyelitis usually involves the metatarsals and phalanges (and calcaneum). Gout must often be considered; urate is a negative acute-phase reactant and its being normal does not exclude acute gout! However, this appearance is not suggestive and gout does not explain the neuropathic findings or plasma glucose.

The main problem is misdiagnosing Charcot's as osteomyelitis or gout. Thus a high index of suspicion for Charcot's is necessary. Once it is diagnosed the principal treatment is total abstinence from putting weight on the foot till warmth, swelling and redness subside.

Acromegaly causes the following effects on the mature skeleton:

- Increase in both the anterior-posterior and transverse dimensions of the vertebrae
- Widening of the phalanges and tufting of the terminal phalanges
- Widening of the metacarpophalangeal joints due to cartilage hypertrophy
- Osteoarthritis and chondrocalcinosis
- Increased soft-tissue thickness, eg heel pad > 25 mm
- Enlargement of the pituitary fossa with erosion of the floor
- Prognathism
- Enlarged paranasal air sinuses and mastoids
- Enlargement of the occipital protuberance.

There is an established complication of diabetes with the elevated plasma glucose sufficient to diagnose diabetes mellitus. Secondary diabetes occurs in acromegaly and in Cushing's syndrome.

Case 20

1   A   Cushing's syndrome

2   G   Midnight cortisol
     J   Low-dose dexamethasone suppression test

She has diabetes (possibly secondary diabetes) and hypertension. The lipids are typical of the metabolic syndrome. The clinical image shows moon facies, supraclavicular fat pads, central obesity, thin limbs, bruises and purple striae. These are the features of Cushing's syndrome and this is the likely diagnosis. The appropriate next step is confirmation of the suspected diagnosis. There are a large number of options at this stage, but of these choices, the best approach would be to perform a standard 48-hour low-dose dexamethasone suppression test and augment the sensitivity of this approach by performing a midnight cortisol.

The glucose tolerance is not normal; the allusion to normality is the normal fasting plasma glucose, but the patient is on treatment and the HbA_{1c} is high. To get this wrong would be unforgivable.

Cushing's disease refers to a specific aetiology of Cushing's syndrome, ie pituitary-dependent. Haemochromatosis is unlikely as she is still menstruating.

Rosiglitazone-induced hepatitis is a possibility but there is not enough information to make this diagnosis; it is more likely that she has a degree of non-alcoholic steatohepatitis as part of the metabolic syndrome.

Stopping or increasing the rosiglitazone, stopping both (and starting insulin), or measuring a serum ferritin are all reasonable answers but are not the best answer. (This is often the case in MRCP; the marks are only there for the **best** answer.) ERCP, liver biopsy or MRI pituitary are not reasonable at this stage. MRI pituitary would potentially be reasonable when considering the aetiology of Cushing's. She does not have a high enough risk to warrant a statin with her age and blood pressure and not being a smoker.

Case 21

1   **D**   Measure growth hormone during an oral glucose tolerance test
     E   Pituitary MRI

The hand is broad, squared and spadelike and is that of a patient with acromegaly. The diagnostic test is to measure growth hormone during a 75-g oral glucose tolerance test. In health it should suppress to be undetectable after a glucose load – most assays should set their detection limit at 0.5 mU/L (0.25 ng/mL). The oral glucose tolerance test must be augmented by measuring the serum IGF-I and comparing it with the age and sex normal range.

Once acromegaly has been diagnosed one should consider the aetiology. Benign pituitary tumours are by far the commonest cause of acromegaly, though rarely carcinoma may be responsible. In up to 10% of cases the pituitary adenoma may be associated with other endocrine tumours, as in multiple endocrine neoplasia – the most common are parathyroid tumours resulting in primary hyperparathyroidism.

Carcinoid tumours, usually of the pancreas or lung, may rarely cause acromegaly by secreting growth hormone-releasing hormone. These patients have somatotroph hyperplasia rather than adenomas, which nonetheless will enlarge the fossa.

The pituitary should therefore be imaged and the correct method is with an MRI unless there is a contraindication. A skull or pituitary X-ray may show an enlarged fossa, but it is too crude and of course will not show small tumours.

The mean of the growth hormone day-curve is useful to assess the activity of the disease once diagnosed.

An insulin tolerance test is the gold standard for assessing growth hormone reserve where deficiency is suspected.

On a foot X-ray one may see an increased heel pad thickness in acromegaly (see p. 177).

Case 22

1   D   Hyperparathyroidism

The X-ray shows resorption of the terminal tufts of the phalanges; subperiosteal bone resorption is the earliest radiological sign and is specific for hyperparathyroidism. Generalised demineralisation is a later finding. Bone disease is now seen in only 10% of cases of primary hyperparathyroidism – partly due to the increasing routine measurement of serum calcium the disease is picked up at a much earlier stage. Parathyroid bone disease is also seen in advanced renal failure – when the GFR gets below about 25 mL/min – when it can be due to either secondary or tertiary hyperparathyroidism.

Subperiosteal bone resorption classically involves the phalanges but can involve other sites, including the outer ends and under-surfaces of the clavicles, the metaphyses of growing ends of long bones, the ischial tuberosities, the symphysis pubis, sacroiliac joints and inner wall of the dorsum sellae. Brown tumours sometimes occur in primary hyperparathyroidism but are less common in secondary hyperparathyroidism. Pathologically, 60% of patients with primary hyperparathyroidism have renal calculi or nephrocalcinosis but the radiological demonstration of this is far less common. Generalised demineralisation can be observed in the skull where it results in a 'pepper pot' appearance. (See also p. 176.)

Nocturia, which is often an early manifestation of diabetes – whether mellitus or insipidus – is a consequence of hypercalcaemia; this is probably due to down-regulation of aquaporin-2 channels in the distal collecting tubule.

Diabetic cheiroarthropathy and acromegaly are dealt with elsewhere (see Book 3, 4.16, and p. 178, respectively).

Osteomalacia is a cause of generalised demineralisation but the major radiological features are stress fractures or pseudofractures – Looser's zones.

Case 23

1   **B**   Multiple myeloma

He is breathless commensurate with his anaemia, possibly compounded by a degree of chronic obstructive pulmonary disease (the hemidiaphragms are flattened and the lungs are over-inflated). He has been treated for several infections and this suggests immunosuppression, which may be caused by:

- Immunosuppressive drugs:
    glucocorticoids
    ciclosporin
    azathioprine
    cyclophosphamide
- Malignancy:
    lymphoma
    chronic lymphocytic leukaemia
- Immunoglobulin deficiency:
    myeloma
    nephrotic syndrome
    protein-losing enteropathy
- HIV infection/AIDS
- Diabetes mellitus.

NB many specific infections are more common, some almost exclusive and several more severe with more severe complications in diabetes mellitus; however the feeling that infection is *more* common is not backed up by very strong evidence.

The only diagnosis that can explain a normochromic anaemia, mild neutropenia, thrombocytopenia, renal failure, hypoalbuminaemia, and highly elevated globulins is myeloma. The X-ray shows several lytic lesions, best seen in the left humerus. They are punched-out with no sclerotic margin and would be consistent with multiple myeloma or, less likely, multiple secondaries. The alkaline phosphatase is usually normal in myeloma unless there has been a pathological fracture; in secondaries it is usually elevated.

Most patients (98%) have a monoclonal protein either in the serum, urine, or both, and so electrophoresis and immunoglobulin levels ought to be performed. The normal immunoglobulins are depressed. Bence-Jones protein is poorly detected on dipstick tests. Bence Jones proteinuria occurs in only two-thirds of cases; urine should be sent to the lab for detection ± quantification of Bence Jones protein.

At this stage a haematologist should be consulted, the bone marrow examined, β_2-microglobulin measured and a skeletal survey performed.

Milk alkali is rarely seen with ingestion of large amounts of calcium containing alkalis for 'indigestion'. The X-ray does not show a primary lung cancer. The biochemistry of hyperparathyroidism and the hypercalcaemia associated with squamous cell carcinoma (PTHrp) are broadly identical (see also Book 3, 1.12).

Case 24

1   C   Pituitary MRI

TSH-secreting pituitary tumours are rare, and are historically under-diagnosed. In primary hyperthyroidism the TSH should be undetectable; on a modern assay if it is detectable it implies something is amiss and must be followed up. There is no doubt about the free hormone levels as the patient is clinically thyrotoxic. The details tell you that the thyroid function has already been repeated and was abnormal on another assay.

The first cause that must be considered is antibody interference. One would normally ask the lab to send the sample away to be assayed with different antibodies to negate the presence of heterophile antibodies; these are present in ~0.05% of the population and can interfere with immunoassays. These thyroid function tests are abnormal at two hospitals, implying assay interference is not the problem.

The diagnosis to exclude is a thyrotroph adenoma. If there is any suggestion of a large pituitary mass, visual fields must be performed clinically without delay and if this suggests optic chiasm compression, a scan of the pituitary must follow at the first opportunity. A pituitary image is the first step in establishing the diagnosis; thyrotrophinomas are often macroadenomas. The other means to establish the diagnosis include measurement of α-subunit, TRH, a TRH test and octreotide scanning. The main differential diagnosis is partial pituitary resistance to thyroid hormone.

Free hormone levels are not affected by pregnancy like total hormone assays. Urine β-HCG has the same sensitivity as serum β-HCG (**NB** the latter is also susceptible to heterophile antibodies).

Case 25

1   B   Haemochromatosis

The only answer that can explain diabetes mellitus, atrial fibrillation, arthropathy, tanned skin, hepatosplenomegaly and liver dysfunction – mild hyperbilirubinaemia, transaminitis, synthetic failure – is haemochromatosis. Haemochromatosis has a striking male preponderance because women are protected from iron overload by menstruation. It most commonly presents in middle age. 'Bronzed diabetes' helps one remember the major clinical features. The pigmentation is hypermelanotic. Diabetes, due to pancreatic iron deposition, can be present many years before the other clinical features are evident. Arthritis affecting the knees and metacarpophalangeal joints can be a presenting feature and is associated with calcium pyrophosphate deposition in affected joints (see Book 3, 4.23). Hypogonadism occurs due to iron deposition in both the pituitary and gonads. Hepatomegaly is to be expected whereas splenomegaly is unusual. Cirrhosis and subsequent hepatocellular carcinoma occur. Cardiac arrhythmias and failure occur due to iron deposition.

Haemochromatosis can occur with totally normal liver function and predate diabetes; thus it must be considered to be diagnosed. Serum ferritin, total iron and transferrin saturation are raised and TIBC reduced; there is not a clear cut-off, but a ferritin of $\geqslant 200$ µg/L would stimulate iron studies in this author's mind and a transferrin saturation of > 60% with no apparent cause ought to make one consider liver biopsy. (**NB** Ferritin does not correlate exactly with body iron so if the disease is suspected check the transferrin saturation and consider referral to someone with an interest in the condition.) It is an autosomal recessive disease, linked to HLA A3, caused by a mutation in the *HFE* gene at 6q21.3. The gene frequency in the European population is 1:10 and population studies have revealed both homozygosity and clinically significant iron overload in ~1:300 of the population. If it is picked up early the sequelae are totally preventable, including diabetes, arthritis, hypogonadism, cirrhosis and hepatocellular carcinoma.

The patient has cirrhosis, but it is unreasonable to ascribe this to alcohol here; the liver damage in haemochromatosis is more severe in alcohol users. The drugs are not responsible for all these features – metformin, pioglitazone and simvastatin should all, however, be discontinued; paracetamol can be used in small doses and NSAIDs are associated with an increased risk of gastrointestinal haemorrhage.

Case 26

1 A Elevated renin, normal anion gap acidosis, hyperkalaemia, high TSH

The image shows calcified adrenals. These occur in tuberculous adrenalitis which causes Addison's disease. The biochemical features of this are:

- Hyponatraemia, hyperkalaemia and elevated urea – but only if severely unwell
- Acidosis – normal anion gap
- Hypercalcaemia – rarely

- Hypoglycaemia
- Cortisol can be low, undetectable or normal
- ACTH – always elevated; a suspicion of Addison's is a definite indication for this test
- Renin – always elevated
- T_4 and TSH – may be typical of primary hypothyroidism but return to normal with glucocorticoid treatment.

The biochemistry can be entirely normal, and pigmentation can be obscured by vitiligo or just absent, so a high degree of clinical suspicion is required.

The other answers would be compatible with:

- Hyperparathyroidism (B)
- Hyper-reninaemic hyperaldosteronism, eg renal artery stenosis (C)
- Proximal RTA with hypophosphataemic rickets, eg Fanconi's syndrome (D)
- Phaeochromocytoma – hypokalaemia can be mild (E).

Case 27

1   C   Cushing's disease

The low-dose dexamethasone suppression test is used in some centres as the primary screening and diagnostic test for Cushing's – here it does not show suppression – suggesting Cushing's with about 95% specificity. The high-dose suppression test attempts to elucidate the aetiology. It is important to know the plasma ACTH at this stage – but as is so often the case in the real world, the ACTH is not available with the same rapidity as the cortisol. In adrenal causes there is complete resistance to the effects of exogenous steroids; thus we would expect no suppression. In ectopic ACTH there is no or minimal suppression after exogenous cortisol. In Cushing's disease there is usually a greater than 50% reduction in cortisol after high-dose dexamethasone. Thus Cushing's disease (pituitary-dependent) is the most likely diagnosis.

ACTH-dependent causes account for about 80% of spontaneous Cushing's syndrome, and roughly 80% of these are Cushing's disease and 15% are ectopic ACTH. Of the 20% that are ACTH-independent, 60% are adrenal adenomas and ~40% adrenal carcinomas.

Case 28

1   A   Start aspirin, a standard dose of statin and start an ACE inhibitor and titrate to the maximum dose

This answer can be read in conjunction with the NICE guidelines for the management of type 1 diabetes mellitus (adults).[1]

They have fulfilled the criteria for a diagnosis of microalbuminuria, having two positive screening tests. Urine protein tests are not sensitive enough to pick up the small amounts of albumin and are thus negative. Patients with T1DM should have a screening test for microalbuminuria yearly and if positive it should be repeated in the following weeks. There is no obligation to go on and check a 24-hour albumin excretion but microalbuminuria is defined as a 24-hour albumin excretion of between 30 and 300 mg/day. It is a highly significant finding and confers the highest risk of arterial disease on the patient and as such they should be started on aspirin and a statin. The microalbuminuria dictates treatment with an ACE inhibitor titrated up to the maximum dose (if not tolerated use an angiotensin II-receptor blocker). The blood pressure must be maintained below 130/80 mmHg. One should suspect other renal disease if the blood pressure is significantly raised, proteinuria is sudden, haematuria is present, there is systemic ill health, or in the absence of progressive retinopathy. In that case (depending on local practice) either you or a renal/diabetic clinic ought to investigate further.

This degree of retinopathy away from the macula is background retinopathy and as such can just be observed. One would expect some benefit with ACE inhibition. Many people would refer to an eye clinic for surveillance with retinal photography. Hard exudates or disease near the macula would warrant referral; new vessel formation should be referred for rapid review; sudden loss of vision, rubeosis iridis, pre-retinal or vitreous haemorrhage, or retinal detachment should be referred for emergency review.

[1] http://www.nice.org.uk/pdf/CG015adultsquickrefguide.pdf

Case 29

1   E   Add ezetimibe

His LDL is too high and must be controlled, aiming to bring the total cholesterol down to < 5 mmol/L and the LDL to < 3.0 mmol/L at the least. The triglyceride level of concern according to the current guidelines from NICE is 2.3 mmol/L. What is the best agent to bring this patient's LDL down? The options are colestyramine and ezetimibe. Colestyramine is an anion exchange resin that acts by sequestering bile acids in the lumen of the bowel, preventing their resorption as part of the enterohepatic circulation. This promotes hepatic conversion of cholesterol into bile acids; the resultant increased LDL-receptor activity of liver cells increases the clearance of LDL cholesterol and effectively reduces LDL cholesterol. It can cause problems with hypertriglyceridaemia and so it is not a prudent choice here. Ezetimibe selectively inhibits transport of cholesterol across the lumen of the small intestine, reducing delivery of cholesterol to the liver. It may provide an additional 10% of LDL-lowering additional to statins. It is licensed for this indication, as well as monotherapy alongside appropriate dietary and lifestyle modification.

Fish oils are sometimes useful for severe hypertriglyceridaemia, but can aggravate hypercholesterolaemia. Fibrates are the most potent triglyceride-lowering drugs, but when used with profound hypertriglyceridaemia tend to increase LDL. The nicotinic acid group is the most potent at increasing HDL. They also reduce triglycerides and improve the particle size of LDL; they are limited by flushing. The modified-release formulation and synthetic cousin – acipimox – may reduce this. The class is limited by a lack of comparative evidence.

Case 30

1   **B**   Amiodarone

The key points in the history and examination are the dense hemiparesis, suggesting a total anterior circulation stroke, together with the chaotic pulse: this must make one think of thromboembolic phenomena, perhaps a mural thrombus because of underlying atrial fibrillation? The pulse is only 60 bpm, he is cool, pale and obese, with moderate diastolic hypertension and an impalpable apex, together with evidence of volume contraction – this would all be consistent with hypothyroidism. The haematology and biochemistry are consistent with hypothyroidism. The two images, taken 5 months apart, show coarse reticular interstitial shadowing, predominantly involving the mid and lower zones; there is volume loss. The only thing that can tie all these facts together is the amiodarone treatment for atrial fibrillation causing hypothyroidism and pulmonary fibrosis.

Lithium, primarily used for manic-depressive disorders, can cause a nephrogenic diabetes insipidus. Demeclocycline is used occasionally to treat SIADH.

Case 31

1   **C**   Insulinoma

This history describes Whipple's triad, the occurrence of symptoms associated with hypoglycaemia, a low (albeit glucometer) glucose and a resolution of symptoms when the glucose is returned to normal.

Hypoglycaemia is strictly diagnosed as an arterial glucose of < 2.2 mmol/L in practice venous samples are satisfactory.

Hypoglycaemia is either fasting or non-fasting. The causes of fasting hypoglycaemia are:

- Excess insulin-like activity:
  exogenous insulin – usually obvious
  endogenous insulin:
    insulinoma
    sulphonylureas
  insulin-like peptides, eg pro-IGF-II in mesenchymal tumours
- Non-insulin-induced hepatic dysfunction:
  alcohol
  liver failure
  primary or sedondary adrenal failure
  growth hormone deficiency
  inborn errors of metabolism
  severe starvation or severe, excessive exercise.

Non-fasting hypoglycaemia is uncommon.

Urine ketones are absent, indicating excess insulin-like activity suppressing ketogenesis. During the 72-hour fast hypoglycaemia occurs (β-hydroxybutyrate can be taken to furthur gauge insulin activity). While hypoglycaemic, the insulin is detectable, whereas it should be suppressed. This does not differentiate between an insulinoma, exogenous insulin or sulphonylurea/repa/nate-glinide administration. The presence of C peptide demonstrates that it is endogenous insulin (as C peptide is cleaved off from pro-insulin before release); the absence of sulphonylureas or 'glinides' makes an insulinoma the likely diagnosis.

Insulinomas are slow-growing tumours – in retrospect the median time from symptoms to diagnosis is 5 years. About 90% are < 2 cm and 40% are < 1 cm. More than 80% are solitary, 10% are malignant and about 5% are part of MEN 1.

For the purposes of MRCP, the first abnormality in MEN 1 is primary hyperparathyroidism and this is always present unless surgery has been performed. Pancreatic tumours occur in three-quarters, pituitary tumours occur in around a third, prolactin-secreting more commonly than growth hormone. The growth hormone and cortisol are normal during hypoglycaemia – the patient has effectively had an insulin tolerance test with their own insulin.

Chapter Three   Answers

Case 1

1   **D**   Colonoscopy

The symptoms and investigation results are not suggestive of a flare-up of ulcerative colitis and so treatment aimed at treating this would be inappropriate. The most important diagnosis to exclude is colorectal carcinoma.

Chronic inflammatory bowel disease affecting the colon increases the risk of colorectal cancer. This is as true for Crohn's colitis as it is for ulcerative colitis, for which the risk is ~18% after 30 years of disease; the risk increases from practically zero at 8–10 years, by 0.5–1% per year thereafter. Colorectal neoplasia is more likely to develop in patients with pancolitis than in those with left-sided disease, while the risk for those with proctitis is thought to be negligible. The degree of histological inflammation has also recently been shown to be a risk factor. Data are beginning to emerge to suggest that 5-ASA drugs may protect against the risk of developing cancer. Whether this putative effect is related to an associated decrease in chronic inflammation in those on 5-ASA drugs, or is due to other mechanisms is, as yet, uncertain.

Current UK guidelines advise surveillance after 10 years for patients with pancolitis, and after 15–20 years for those with left-sided disease. Thereafter the screening interval is decreased such that patients have colonoscopies 3-yearly after a decade of disease, 2-yearly after 20 years and yearly after 30 years. Patients who also have primary sclerosing cholangitis represent a group at particularly high risk and are therefore screened yearly from diagnosis.

It should be borne in mind that surveillance has not been shown to decrease mortality and that newer, less invasive methods of screening may be employed in the future. Currently, however, mucosal sampling along the entire colon is required to assess for pre-malignant changes and endoscopic screening therefore remains the gold standard.

Case 2

1   **E**   Acute hepatitis E

The picture is of an acute hepatitis; given the history of travel and the lack of other risk factors, the most likely candidate – were it not for the antibodies – would be hepatitis A. This is the most common form of viral hepatitis infection worldwide. It is passed by the faeco-oral route and is hence common in areas with poor sanitation. It has a 2-week incubation period followed by about 2 weeks of nausea and anorexia. Many people infected with the virus then recover spontaneously, but a proportion go on to develop jaundice, at which point they often start to feel better. Rarely, fulminant hepatitis develops; however, there is no chronic or carrier state. IgM antibodies develop about 3 weeks after infection and disappear by about 8 weeks. IgG antibodies appear after 4–5 weeks.

Given that hepatitis C rarely causes an acute hepatitis, and that the patient does not appear to have any risk factors for blood-borne hepatitis viruses, the most likely diagnosis is hepatitis E.

Hepatitis E is, like hepatitis A, an RNA virus. It is also spread via the faeco-oral route and causes a similar picture to hepatitis A virus infection. The risk of fulminant hepatitis is higher with hepatitis E than with hepatitis A: mortality rates for hepatitis A are about 0.5%, whereas for hepatitis E they are 1–2%. Pregnant women are, however, at much higher risk of death from hepatitis E-related hepatic failure, with mortality rates of 10–20%. Treatment, as for hepatitis A, is supportive.

Case 3

1 B Ventilation–perfusion scan

The sudden onset of her symptoms, with a lack of findings in her chest, points toward a thromboembolic event as the cause of her symptoms. A ventilation–perfusion scan is, therefore, the most likely of these tests to establish the diagnosis.

Patients with inflammatory bowel disease (IBD) are at increased risk of thromboembolic events and are about three times as likely to have either a PE or a DVT as healthy controls. Although the risk is higher in patients with active disease, those with inactive disease also have an increased risk. Along with dehydration, hospitalisation and the need to undergo surgery, IBD is also associated with other risk factors for thromboembolism, such as thrombocytosis and increased platelet activation.

D-dimer levels are less likely to be helpful in patients with IBD as they are elevated in active disease. Methotrexate is associated with pulmonary toxicity, although this has never been reported in a patient with IBD and is more likely to have an indolent presentation. IBD is also associated with a number of pulmonary manifestations, including bronchiectasis, bronchitis, organising pneumonia and granulomatous lung disease. These associations are, however, rare in comparison with thromboembolic disease.

Case 4

1   **A**   Autoimmune hepatitis

About 70% of patients with autoimmune hepatitis are female, mostly between the ages of 15 and 40. Non-specific symptoms, such as rashes, malaise, arthralgia and anorexia, may precede jaundice by many months, although the onset of the disease can be abrupt.

Diagnosis is made by a combination of liver biopsy and blood tests. AST levels are normally elevated 2–20 times normal levels. In contrast, an elevated ALP should raise the possibility of primary biliary cirrhosis. About 80% of patients have polyclonal elevation of IgG. The majority of patients have anti-nuclear or anti-smooth muscle antibodies (type 1), or anti-liver/kidney microsomal antibodies (type 2), the latter usually only occurring in children. A minority (10%) also have anti-mitochondrial antibodies. Autoimmune hepatitis can be associated with other autoimmune conditions, such as thyroid disease, vitiligo, type 1 diabetes or Sjögren's syndrome.

Initial treatment with corticosteroids is often supplemented with azathioprine, thereby allowing the dose of steroid to be reduced. Other agents, such as mycophenolate mofetil or tacrolimus, are occasionally used if azathioprine is ineffective. The aim of treatment is to normalise liver function tests, although about a third of patients are cirrhotic when diagnosed. Liver transplantation may be required due to decompensation or to control the complications of cirrhosis.

Case 5

1   **D**   Duodenal ulcer

The angiogram shows contrast in the duodenum, lateral to the midline. In view of her age and history of non-steroidal anti-inflammatory drug usage, she is most likely to have a duodenal ulcer. Although angiography is not commonly used to diagnose upper gastrointestinal bleeding, in some situations it can be useful. Likewise, particularly in patients unlikely to survive laparotomy, it is possible to embolise the source of bleeding when endoscopic treatment is not possible.

Primary aortoenteric fistulae (PAEF) are rare. Fistulation usually occurs into the third or fourth part of the duodenum. Although bleeding can be catastrophic, PAEF usually presents with herald bleeds. Diagnosis is best made by endoscopy and CT scanning. Treatment is surgical. More commonly, fistulation between the aorta and the gastrointestinal tract occurs after aortic surgery and is usually associated with aneurysms.

Bleeding from the oesophagus, be it related to varices or a carcinoma, should be seen in the midline.

Meckel's diverticulum is an embryonic remnant present in about 2% of the population. Complications, including bleeding, inflammation and intussusception, occur in the minority, normally before adulthood. Classically they are said to be twice as common in males as females, two feet from the ileocaecal valve and two inches in length. They can contain two sorts of ectopic tissue – gastric and pancreatic: the so-called rule of twos. Tc-99m scintigraphy can reveal a focus suprapubically, slightly to the right of midline.

Case 6

1   **C**   Duodenal carcinoma

He has a duodenal carcinoma presenting with iron deficiency as part of the familial adenomatous polyposis (FAP) syndrome. FAP was formerly known as familial polyposis coli, but was sensibly renamed as it became apparent that the polyps were not confined to the colon. It causes carpeting of the colon with adenomatous polyps which invariably undergo malignant change, often in early adulthood. It is inherited autosomal dominantly, with complete penetrance. Carriers of an *APC* gene mutation are advised to have prophylactic colectomy.

Although duodenal polyps were first noted in association with FAP over 100 years ago, they have only become an important cause of morbidity and mortality with the development of prophylactic colectomy and its resultant decrease in colorectal carcinoma. The majority of patients with FAP will develop duodenal adenomatous polyps and the risk of duodenal carcinoma is vastly increased compared with the general population: in a recent study, the incidence was about 5% at 57 years of age. Accordingly, screening of the upper gastrointestinal tract is now routine for patients with FAP.

Desmoids are benign tumours that occur in 10–20% of people with FAP. They can occur within the abdomen or abdominal wall but more frequently present with pain than with iron deficiency.

Colectomy should not cause malabsorption of either iron or vitamin B_{12}. Pernicious anaemia causes a macrocytic picture (due to malabsorption of vitamin B_{12}) and is not, in any case, associated with FAP.

Case 7

1   **E**   Distal duodenal biopsy

Despite the absence of anti-endomysial antibodies (EMA), the most important diagnosis to exclude is coeliac disease. About 3% of patients with coeliac disease have selective IgA deficiency and, since EMA tests are for IgA, a proportion of patients with coeliac disease will have false-negative tests. The gold standard in diagnosing coeliac disease remains the response of small-bowel histology to a gluten-free diet. In addition, small-bowel histology may allow the diagnosis of other small-bowel enteropathies.

IgG anti-tissue transglutaminase antibodies and IgG EMA overcome the problem of selective IgA deficiency but, unlike IgA EMA, they are not helpful in assessing the response to a gluten-free diet; IgA EMA disappear following abstinence from gluten.

Case 8

1   E   Gastric carcinoma

The picture is of acanthosis nigricans (AN). It consists of thickening and hyperpigmentation of the skin of the entire body, but especially in flexural areas. AN is associated with insulin resistance; when it occurs *de novo* in the elderly it is more commonly associated with malignancy. Very rarely it is inherited as a Mendelian dominant. Finally, it can be drug-induced – nicotinic acid, diethylstilbestrol, oral contraceptives and exogenous glucocorticoids have all been incriminated. When associated with malignancy, AN presents before the malignancy in a third of patients, with the malignancy in a third, and after malignancy in a third. Although AN has been described in association with many different cancers, when associated with a malignancy it is most commonly a gastrointestinal adenocarcinoma. Of these, gastric carcinoma predominates. The lesions have been known to disappear with treatment of the underlying malignancy and, similarly, can reappear with a recurrence.

AN may occur anywhere, but most commonly appears in the flexural regions – the axillae, groin, and on the posterior surface of the neck. Lesions progress from hyperpigmented macules to palpable plaques. AN is usually asymptomatic but it can cause pruritus.

Unfortunately, it is not possible to distinguish between malignant and non-malignant AN: the former must always be considered, particularly if found in association with suggestive symptoms.

Case 9

1   E   Bile-salt malabsorption

The entirely normal investigations are not suggestive of an inflammatory cause for her diarrhoea, or of small-bowel malabsorption, and the length of the history goes against an infective cause. In fact, her symptoms are more suggestive of idiopathic bile-salt malabsorption. This is often overlooked as a cause of diarrhoea: perhaps as many as a third of patients diagnosed as having irritable bowel syndrome actually have idiopathic bile-salt malabsorption.

Bile acid-related diarrhoea can have other causes: terminal ileal disease or resection can prevent reabsorption of bile acids, and bile-salt malabsorption can also be seen after cholecystectomy. Diagnosis is best made by measuring retention of SeHCAT, a cholic acid derivative combined with radioactive selenium. An alternative is to give a trial of treatment with a bile-salt sequestrant, such as colestyramine. The response to this can be dramatic and patients often have to titrate their dose.

Case 10

1   **A**   Tuberculosis

The changes are classically those of miliary TB, namely, small ~3–4-mm, evenly sized, widely distributed nodular shadows throughout the lung fields. Although sarcoidosis can present with these changes, the nodules are normally larger and have a greater variation in size. Miliary metastases (as opposed to primary lung cancer) tend to be larger and are often fewer in number. Atypical pneumonia can rarely present like this. Taken overall, both the history and X-ray are highly suggestive of miliary TB.

Infliximab is a mouse–human chimeric monoclonal antibody against human tumour necrosis factor-α that has been available for use in the UK since 1999. Controlled trials have shown that it is able to induce remission in active Crohn's disease and can heal Crohn's fistulae.

As with all drugs that have an immunosuppressive effect, there are concerns regarding the safety of infliximab: a particular worry is that infliximab may allow dormant tuberculosis to reactivate. Infliximab-related TB is, in fact, normally extrapulmonary and is now of such concern that patients are screened for TB prior to receiving infliximab. Other infections, including bacterial and fungal infections, have also been reported in association with infliximab therapy.

Other side effects described in association with infliximab include infusion reactions, the development of antibodies, demyelinating syndromes, and possibly a long-term risk of malignancy. As yet, however, no link with malignancy has been established.

Case 11

1   B   Oesophageal carcinoma

The barium swallow shows an oesophageal carcinoma. The incidence of oesophageal carcinoma is rising. It occurs more commonly in men than in women (4:1) and squamous cell carcinomas, which are more commonly in the upper or mid-oesophagus, outnumber adenocarcinomas (normally distal) 3 to 1. Risk factors for squamous cell carcinomas include smoking and alcohol, while adenocarcinomas normally occur in association with Barrett's oesophagus.

Staging requires CT scanning, ideally in combination with endoscopic ultrasound, which is the best modality for assessing local invasion and hence suitability for resection. Chemoradiation is the treatment of choice for localised proximal squamous carcinoma. Otherwise, chemotherapy and radiotherapy, in combination or alone, have some role in the management of oesophageal carcinoma.

Dilation at first presentation is inappropriate for potentially operable tumours and, although sometimes used later in the disease, carries a higher risk of perforation than for benign tumours. Dysphagia is often best treated with endoscopically inserted expandable metal stents. These, however, may not improve dysphagia if symptoms are minimal. Alternative palliative treatments for dysphagia include alcohol injection and laser therapy.

Case 12

1   C   *Giardia lamblia*

The symptoms are those of giardiasis. *Giardia* is a flagellated protozoan found worldwide, although it is particularly common in developing countries. Spread of infection is usually water-borne (potentially causing epidemics) or by direct faeco-oral transmission. Ingestion of cysts leads to trophozoite infestation of the small intestine.

About 60% of people will have no symptoms and will simply carry the infection, excreting cysts. Of those who develop symptoms, the majority develop watery diarrhoea 1–2 weeks after ingestion of cysts and some will go on to develop malabsorption, which may be profound. Other symptoms include nausea, flatulence, bloating and anorexia.

Diagnosis is made by examination of the stool for cysts and trophozoites, although negative stools do not exclude the diagnosis: parasites are excreted at irregular intervals. Accordingly, it is common practice to colect serial stools for examination. Duodenal aspirates and specific antibodies may be helpful.

Treatment is with metronidazole or tinidazole, but it is not uncommon to need repeated courses to eliminate the infection.

Entamoeba histolytica causes colitis as does *Balantidium coli*. *Entamoeba coli* is normally non-pathogenic and *Cryptosporidium parvum* normally causes a self-limiting watery diarrhoeal illness lasting 7–10 days. In immunocompromised hosts, however, *C. parvum*-related diarrhoea can be much more severe.

Case 13

1   B   Hepatocellular carcinoma (HCC)

Given the patient's racial origin and the α-feto protein (AFP) level, the diagnosis is likely to be hepatitis B-related HCC. An elevated AFP level occurs in 80% of patients with HCC, although other tumours, such as testicular, ovarian and pancreatic tumours, can rarely cause raised AFP levels. Diagnosis is based on a combination of clinical suspicion, AFP levels and radiological findings. Biopsy of potentially operable lesions is discouraged by some due to the risk of tumour seeding.

HCC normally occurs as a complication of cirrhosis which, on a worldwide basis, is most commonly due to hepatitis B. Screening cirrhotic patients with regular AFP testing and ultrasound examination of the liver is potentially a huge healthcare burden, but is increasingly practised.

Early HCC can be resected, although this requires reasonable liver function. Liver transplantation is also feasible for early disease. Otherwise, radiofrequency ablation, embolisation, chemoembolisation and alcohol instillation are all used with varying success.

Although CA 125 is a tumour marker for ovarian cancer, levels are also increased in the presence of ascites.

Case 14

1   C   HELLP syndrome

HELLP syndrome (Haemolysis, Elevated Liver enzymes and Low Platelets) normally occurs in the third trimester of pregnancy, although it can present in the second trimester or post-partum. Clotting abnormalities are not usually present unless disseminated intravascular coagulation develops and hypertension is not universally seen. HELLP syndrome is more common in white, multiparous women over the age of 25 and can recur in subsequent pregnancies. By contrast, risk factors for pre-eclampsia, which is far more common, include first pregnancy, extremes of reproductive age, family history of pre-eclampsia, chronic hypertension and multiple gestation. HELLP syndrome can co-exist with pre-eclampsia.

Management depends on the gestational age of the fetus, if presentation is before 32 weeks then conservative management, in a centre experienced with dealing with HELLP, combined with corticosteroid administration to encourage fetal lung development, may be appropriate. Should deterioration occur, then delivery is indicated. If presentation is after 34 weeks gestation then the fetus should be delivered. Management of hypertension, if present, is indicated and platelet transfusions may be required.

Hyperemesis gravidarum is characterised by nausea and vomiting persisting beyond the 14th week of pregnancy.

Intrahepatic cholestasis of pregnancy is a self-limiting condition occurring in the third trimester. It is usually preceded by pruritus.

Acute fatty liver of pregnancy also presents in the third trimester, typically with nausea, abdominal pain and encephalopathy. It can be fatal without prompt delivery.

Case 15

1   **B**   Propranolol

Variceal haemorrhage carries with it a significant mortality. The risk of death is closely related to the severity of liver disease. If variceal haemorrhage is suspected, upper gastrointestinal endoscopy should be carried out at the earliest opportunity once the patient has been resuscitated. This allows not only confirmation of the diagnosis, but also the opportunity to control bleeding; variceal band ligation or sclerotherapy are the two treatments most commonly used.

Terlipressin is a synthetic vasopressin analogue that causes splanchnic vasoconstriction and, subsequently, a drop in portal pressure. It is particularly useful when endoscopy is unavailable and has been shown to decrease bleeding and improve survival.

Variceal haemorrhage is commonly associated with bacterial infections, the presence of which affect outcome adversely. Trials have shown that prophylactic antibiotics are successful in decreasing infection rates and also improve short-term survival. Typically, fluoroquinolones are used, although other antibiotic combinations may be effective.

All patients with ascites complicating cirrhosis should have a diagnostic peritoneal tap. The diagnosis of spontaneous bacterial peritonitis should always be sought and, once made, is an indication to consider referral for liver transplantation. However, continued abuse of alcohol must be addressed if transplantation is considered.

Although beta-blockade is an important part of primary and secondary prevention of variceal haemorrhage, it is inappropriate in the initial management of an unstable patient.

Case 16

1   **A**   Mesalazine
    B   Stop smoking
    C   Stop ibuprofen

He has a terminal ileal stricture, likely to be due to Crohn's disease (CD). Smoking is known not only to predispose to CD but also to affect disease outcome adversely. All patients with CD should be encouraged to stop smoking. Mesalazine, in a preparation that delivers the drug to the small bowel, is an appropriate first-line treatment for active CD if the patient is well. Many patients will, however, require steroids at some point. Immunosuppressive drugs are also an important part of the armoury of medical treatments for CD but are not generally used first-line, particularly in relatively well patients. Infliximab is relatively contraindicated in patients with stricturing CD as it can induce rapid healing and bowel obstruction.

Loperamide is often used as an antidiarrhoeal in CD but should be avoided in patients in whom active colonic involvement is suspected (as in this case, as indicated by bloody diarrhoea) as it may predispose to colonic dilatation. Non-steroidal anti-inflammatory drugs can exacerbate inflammatory bowel disease in some patients and should probably be avoided if possible.

Surgery is an important part of management of CD and may be an extremely effective treatment, for example, in patients with limited ileal disease. In patients who are well, with minimal symptoms, a trial of medical therapy is warranted.

Elemental diets are an alternative treatment but, perhaps due to their palatability, are more commonly used in children than in adults.

Ileal tuberculosis, particularly in patients from endemic areas, should be considered as a differential diagnosis and can present identically to this. This may make steroids less likely to be used as a first-line drug here, particularly as the patient is well, at least until biopsies have been taken. CD, overall remains more likely.

Case 17

1   A   Referral to the surgical team for laparotomy

The X ray shows Rigler's sign. Both sides of the bowel wall can be identified (one example arrowed), indicating free air within the peritoneal cavity. Successful management requires a laparotomy.

Any form of infectious colitis can result in perforation, although this is a rare complication. Given the history of dysentery and travel to Asia, amoebiasis, enterohaemorrhagic *Escherichia coli, Shigella* spp. and *Salmonella* spp. should be considered.

Salmonella typhi can cause terminal ileal perforation due to necrosis of Peyer's patches. Risk factors for perforation include male sex, a short duration of symptoms and leucopenia.

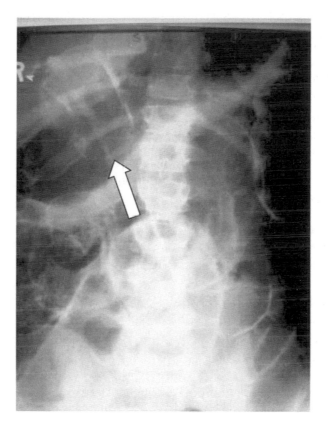

Case 18

1   **D**   pH 7.25

Paracetamol overdosage is the most common form of self-poisoning encountered and can be fatal. The decision of whether to treat with the antidote N-acetylcysteine (NAC) is based on the plasma levels of paracetamol and the time since the overdose was taken. A nomogram for patients at normal risk and those at high risk (such as patients on enzyme-inducing drugs, the malnourished, the alcohol-dependent or those who drank alcohol with the overdose is available in the *BNF*[1]. If a potentially toxic dose of paracetamol has been taken (7.5 g), treatment should be initiated prior to the results of paracetamol levels becoming available.

Unfortunately, some patients present after 16 hours, after which time the value of plasma paracetamol levels is questionable. However, there is good evidence for the use of NAC in such cases. In patients in whom liver failure does not develop, decisions about psychiatric assessment must be made prior to discharge.

Predicting the outcome of patients who have paracetamol-related liver failure in the early stages of the disease is not easy. As deterioration can be rapid, it is important to consider referral to a liver transplant unit early. Recent guidelines, shown below, outline the criteria for referral to such a unit[2].

Day 2	Day 3	Day 4
Arterial pH < 7.30	Arterial pH < 7.30	
INR > 3	INR > 4	Any rise in INR
Encephalopathy	Encephalopathy	Encephalopathy
Creatinine > 200 μmol/L	Creatinine > 200 μmol/L	Creatinine > 250 μmol/L
Hypoglycaemia		

[1] http://www.bnf.org/bnf/bnf/current/openat/
[2] Devlin J, O'Grady J. 1999. Indications for referral and assessment in adult liver transplantation: a clinical guideline. *Gut*, 45 (Suppl 6), VI1–VI22.

Case 19

1   **C**   Pancreatic carcinoma

The ERCP image shows a dilated duct above a stricture in the lower common bile duct. Often, when visualized, the pancreatic duct is also dilated: this is the so-called 'double duct' sign.

The incidence of pancreatic cancer is rising in Europe. It tends to affect men more than women and has a very poor 5-year survival of about 1%

(compared with much better survival rates for ampullary carcinoma).

Cancers in the head of the pancreas tend to present earlier than those in the body or tail. Typically, the former present with obstructive jaundice while the latter cause epigastric pain and weight loss. Risk factors include smoking, chronic pancreatitis, advancing age and diabetes mellitus. Inherited pancreatic cancer syndromes are rare but recognised.

Surgical resection, although potentially curative, is rarely possible, and both chemotherapy and radiotherapy have limited efficacy. Palliation is often all that is possible. Endoscopic or percutaneous relief of obstructive jaundice may be required. Duodenal obstruction is not uncommon and often requires a surgical bypass procedure, although endoscopic stent insertion can sometimes relieve symptoms.

Case 20

1 **A** Erythema nodosum

2 **D** Ulcerative colitis

The lesions shown are erythema nodosum (EN). These tender red nodules normally appear on the extensor surfaces of the lower limbs but can occur elsewhere. It is more commonly found in women (male:female, 1:4) and tends to occur in young adults, although it is found in all age groups. Biopsy of the lesions reveals a panniculitis.

The causes of EN are myriad, such as bacterial infections (including causes of infectious diarrhoea such as *Salmonella* and *Campylobacter*), fungal infections, drugs, pregnancy, lymphoma and sarcoidosis. Inflammatory bowel disease is known to cause EN with a reported incidence of 3–15%. It occurs more commonly in patients with Crohn's disease than in those with ulcerative colitis and is more prevalent in patients with colonic disease. Therapy is aimed at treating the bowel inflammation, although topical symptomatic treatment can be helpful.

Ulcerative colitis can present in any age group but has two peaks of incidence throughout life: most cases present in early adulthood but a second peak occurs later in life. Infective diarrhoea is a well-recognised trigger for ulcerative colitis and should be considered in patients with non-resolving diarrhoea, particularly if it is bloody.

Case 21

1 **E** Treatment with ribavirin

Hepatitis B virus is a blood-borne DNA virus that has infected a significant proportion of the world's population. Carrier rates are higher in the developing world where vertical transmission is more common.

Acute infection is often subclinical and the majority of infected people clear the virus. Persistence of surface antigen suggests chronic infection, while persistence of e antigen implies continued viral replication and high infectivity. Accordingly, family members of such people should be screened for hepatitis B and members of the household who are negative should be vaccinated. Abstinence from alcohol in chronic hepatitis B is advisable as is vaccination against hepatitis A; concurrent hepatitis A could cause liver decompensation.

Treatment of hepatitis B with antiviral drugs is a rapidly developing area. It is important, however, to gauge the degree of inflammation histologically prior to treatment. A particular confounding factor in this instance is the high alcohol intake as some of the transaminase elevation may be related to alcohol. In this case, however, the ALT:AST ratio is suggestive of a viral aetiology rather than an alcoholic one, in which the ratio would be reversed.

Case 22

1   **C**   Achalasia

A fluid level is visible behind the heart and the oesophagus is dilated. This is suggestive of chronic oesophageal obstruction.

Achalasia can present at any age but is rare in childhood. Dysphagia is universal and occurs for liquids and solids relatively early in the condition. Other symptoms include regurgitation, weight loss, pain and aspiration pneumonia, which can be the presenting complaint. Achalasia is caused by degeneration of the myenteric plexus, causing failure of relaxation of the lower oesophageal sphincter (LOS) and absent peristalsis in the body of the oesophagus. Diagnosis is confirmed by oesophageal manometry, but prior upper gastrointestinal endoscopy is mandatory to exclude a tumour of the cardia. Tumours of the cardia can mimic achalasia and chronic achalasia slightly increases the risk of oesophageal carcinoma.

Treatment is either with endoscopic dilatation (which carries the risk of perforation), injection of botulinum toxin into the LOS (which has varying success), or surgical intervention.

Chagas' disease can also mimic achalasia and is caused by *Trypanosoma cruzi*. Chagas' disease, however, is confined to South and Central America.

Case 23

1   **B**   Hydatid disease

Hydatid disease is caused by the ingestion of *Echinococcus granulosus*, a dog tapeworm. It is common in parts of the world associated with raising sheep or cattle, namely the Eastern Mediterranean, South America, the Middle East, Australia, and North and East Africa. The life cycle of *E. granulosus* includes a stage in pigs, cattle or sheep. It is passed to humans by direct contact with dogs or their faeces. Penetration through the duodenal wall permits the parasite passage to the liver from where it can spread to almost any organ. The liver is by far the most common site for hydatid cysts (60%), followed by the lungs (20%).

Hydatid cysts can be asymptomatic but, due to enlarging size, they can cause localised pressure effects such as pain or jaundice. About a third of patients have a peripheral eosinophilia. Complement fixation or haemagglutination tests are often, if not invariably, positive. About 40% of cysts calcify and ultrasound or CT imaging frequently shows daughter cysts.

Many asymptomatic cysts can be left alone. Medical therapy with albendazole can shrink cysts, a measure that is used prior to surgery. Although aspiration was traditionally avoided due to the risk of anaphylaxis, it is now used therapeutically under chemotherapeutic cover. Complications of untreated hydatid disease include involvement of other organs, secondary infection and cyst rupture.

Case 24

1   **A**   Bezoar

The X-ray shows a mass arising from the upper central abdomen. This appears to contain both air and some other material. The rest of the bowel is displaced inferiorly. The mass therefore is likely to be gastric in origin.

Although both duodenal ulceration and gastric malignancy can cause gastric outlet obstruction, for the stomach to enlarge to this size must have taken a considerable period of time. Gastric outflow obstruction tends to present with vomiting before the stomach becomes as dilated as this.

This patient had a bezoar, which when removed was found to weigh 3 kg. Bezoars are concretions of foreign matter within the gastrointestinal tract and are described in many forms including hair (trichobezoar), vegetable matter (phytobezoar) and persimmon. Predisposing factors include ingesting indigestible matter, which may be part of a psychiatric or personality disorder, inadequate chewing, gastric stasis (which may be caused by the bezoar itself and previous gastric surgery. Trichophagia (eating hair) is often found in patients with trichotillomania (compulsive pulling out of hair).

Treatments include enzymatic dissolution of the bezoar, mechanical methods applied endoscopically and laser fragmentation. Larger bezoars, however, often require surgical intervention.

Case 25

1   **D**   Peutz–Jegher syndrome

The history of small-bowel obstruction with the classic signs of perioral pigmentation fits with Peutz–Jegher syndrome. This is a dominantly inherited disorder, the genetic defect being on chromosome 19. The characteristic pigmentation occurs circumorally, on the buccal mucosa, and may also occur on the hands and feet, and around the anus. The pigmented areas may fade with age. Hamartomatous polyps develop, typically in the small intestine, although they can occur in the stomach and colon. Small-intestinal intussusception can lead to small-bowel obstruction requiring laparotomy. Accordingly, once diagnosed, screening for small-intestinal polyps is undertaken. If found proximally, large polyps may be removed endoscopically but, as enteroscopy cannot access the entire length of the small bowel, surgery is often required. Radiological screening of the small bowel may be replaced by capsule endoscopy. Carriers of Peutz–Jegher syndrome are at increased risk of both intestinal and extra-intestinal malignancy.

HHT classically presents with epistaxis at a mean age of 12 years; by 21 years over 90% are manifest. Telangiectasia (rather than pigmented spots) occur on the lips, oral mucosa, tongue (where bleeding can be difficult to control), face, conjunctivae, ears and fingers. Upper gastrointestinal haemorrhage occurs frequently, causing anaemia which often requires transfusion. Other visceral angiodysplasias occur, including pulmonary AVMs, and vascular abnormalities in the liver can lead to cirrhosis.

Cronkhite–Canada syndrome is a very rare disorder characterised by multiple intestinal polyps, alopecia, nail dystrophy and widespread skin pigmentation. It does not appear to have a familial tendency and normally presents with diarrhoea.

Juvenile polyposis can also cause small-intestinal polyps.

FAP is discussed elsewhere (pp. 190; 211).

Case 26

1   **E**   Collagenous colitis

Collagenous colitis predominantly affects women (male:female, 1·4) in the fifth and sixth decades of life. The aetiology is unknown, although an association with non-steroidal anti-inflammatory drugs has been noted. It typically causes chronic watery diarrhoea five to ten times per day, but rarely at night. It is often accompanied by crampy, diffuse abdominal pain and is associated with coeliac disease and other autoimmune disorders. Blood tests are normally unremarkable and both radiological and macroscopic appearances tend to be normal. Diagnosis is made based on the typical histological appearances of a thickened subepithelial collagen band (> 10 microns, normal < 5), a moderate inflammatory cell infiltrate and an increase in intraepithelial lymphocytes. Treatments for collagenous colitis include antidiarrhoeal agents, 5-aminosalicylate drugs, corticosteroids and bile acid sequestrants, all of which are variably effective.

Case 27

1   **B**   Phenobarbital

The picture is of acute pancreatitis. Drugs known to cause pancreatitis include, other than those mentioned the question, azathioprine, furosemide, thiazides, tetracyclines, oestrogens and sulphonamides. Phenobarbital is not known to cause acute pancreatitis.

Amylase levels of more than four times the upper limit of normal are highly suggestive of acute pancreatitis. Factors occurring in the first 48 hours that indicate severe pancreatitis and a poor prognosis include:

- Age   > 55 years
- Blood glucose   > 10 mmol/L
- WCC   > 15.0 × 10^9/L
- Urea   > 16 mmol/L
- Albumin   < 32 g/L
- AST   > 200 U/L
- Calcium   < 2.0 mmol/L
- PO_2 < 8.0 kPa.

Acute severe pancreatitis is often complicated by multiple organ failure and is associated with mortality rates as high as 30%.

Case 28

1   **D**   Pharyngeal pouch

The barium swallow shows a pharyngeal pouch (or Zenker's diverticulum). These occur predominantly in elderly men (male:female, 5:1) and are pulsion diverticula through Killian's dehiscence. They are rare before the age of 40. The aetiology is unclear, though they may be related to poor relaxation of the upper oesophageal sphincter. An association with gastro-oesophageal reflux has also been noted.

Pharyngeal pouches commonly cause dysphagia, regurgitation and aspiration, and are a rare cause of halitosis. If large they can cause a mass in the neck that gurgles on palpation (Boyce's sign).

Regurgitation of the contents of the pouch can ease dysphagia temporarily until the pouch refills with food and fluid. Upper gastrointestinal endoscopy is risky as the pouches are thin-walled and easy to perforate and this is the reason that barium swallows are commonly performed as the first-line investigation in elderly patients with dysphagia. Treatment is surgical with either an open or endoscopic approach.

Schatzki rings are benign narrowings in the distal oesophagus. Post-cricoid webs occur near the upper oesophageal sphincter and can occur in association with iron deficiency anaemia (Patterson– Brown– Kelly syndrome).

Case 29

1   **B**   Recurrent polyserositis (familial Mediterranean fever)

Familial Mediterranean fever (FMF) presents typically, although not exclusively, in Turkish, Armenian, Arabic or Sephardic Jewish people. It is an autosomal recessive disorder, the abnormality being on chromosome 16. About half of patients have no family history of the condition. It typically presents at a young age, with only 5–10% presenting after the age of 20.

FMF is characterised by recurrent episodes of fever with severe abdominal pain and signs of peritonitis, and so patients often have a history of previous surgery, particularly appendectomy. Other commonly described symptoms include pleuritis, pericarditis, synovitis and an erysipeloid rash on the lower limbs. Attacks normally occur without warning and typically last for 24–72 hours. Blood tests are consistent with an acute-phase response. Attacks can normally be prevented with colchicine, which also prevents the development of amyloidosis.

Acute intermittent porphyria, renal colic and abdominal angina do not tend to present with fever.

Case 30

1 **D** Refeeding syndrome

Refeeding syndrome is defined as severe electrolyte and fluid shifts occurring in malnourished patients undergoing refeeding. It is characterised by abnormalities of glucose metabolism and fluid balance, hypophosphataemia, hypomagnesaemia, and hypokalaemia. It can occur with either enteral or parenteral feeding and can be fatal.

Clinical manifestations, if present, are related to the electrolyte and fluid disturbances and are therefore protean. When refeeding syndrome is encountered, electrolyte imbalances can be corrected with intravenous or oral supplementation. Prevention, however, is preferable and graded introduction of calories, along with monitoring of electrolytes before and after the reintroduction of food is advisable. It is also important to consider vitamin deficiencies in such patients, particularly thiamine (vitamin B_1) deficiency which can cause Wernicke's encephalopathy or Korsakoff's syndrome.

Case 31

1 **A** Pyoderma gangrenosum
D Ulcerative colitis

The lesion depicted is pyoderma gangrenosum (PG). Typically, this starts as a small papule or pustule that is often mistaken for an insect bite. This rapidly spreads into an ulcerating lesion with pain being a predominant feature. Although PG can occur at any age, it is most common in the fourth and fifth decades of life. Sex distribution is equal and about half of cases occur in association with a systemic illness. Other than inflammatory bowel disease, PG is commonly associated with arthritides, which may be seropositive or seronegative, and haematological (often malignant) disorders. Less commonly, it is associated with a wide range of disorders, including diverticular disease, liver disease, solid tumours and diabetes mellitus, to name but a few.

Diagnosis is based on histology and clinical findings, and treatment involves the use of topical and systemic corticosteroids, and immunosuppressants.

The barium enema shows the typical 'hosepipe' colon appearance found in chronic ulcerative colitis. Pyoderma gangrenosum was originally thought to be pathognomonic of ulcerative colitis. Incidentally, the patient also has situs inversus.

Case 32

1   D   Sphincter of Oddi dysfunction

The symptoms and response to sphincterotomy are characteristic of sphincter of Oddi dysfunction (SOD). SOD causes non-calculous obstruction of flow of biliary and/or pancreatic fluid. In SOD the sphincter is hypertonic (> 40 mmHg) and can also be dyskinetic. Typically, SOD occurs in middle-aged women but may present in any age group, including children. The presenting symptoms are normally of typical biliary-type pain: it is usually epigastric or right hypochondrial, severe, steady and may radiate to the back or shoulder. Jaundice is rare. Because of the similarity to biliary pain, the diagnosis of SOD is often only made after cholecystectomy. SOD may also cause pancreatitis and it has been suggested that up to a third of cases of idiopathic pancreatitis may be due to SOD.

SOD is divided into three types: type I describes patients with typical biliary pain, abnormal liver enzymes and radiological evidence of impaired biliary drainage; type II describes typical pain with only one of the above two abnormalities; and type III is classified as patients with biliary pain but no other abnormalities. Definitive diagnosis is made by manometry although delayed drainage of contrast is a classic sign at ERCP (> 45 minutes). Rates of post-ERCP pancreatitis are increased five-fold in patients with SOD.

Treatment with smooth-muscle relaxants, such as nifedipine, improves symptoms in a proportion of patients but at approximately placebo rates. Endoscopic sphincterotomy is the current gold standard treatment and is more effective in type I SOD than in types II or III.

Case 33

1   D   Niacin deficiency

The changes are typical of pellagra which is caused by niacin deficiency. Although pellagra is said to present classically with the triad of dementia, dermatitis and diarrhoea, not all of these changes are always present – indeed, constipation can occur. The dermatitis affects sun-exposed areas and progresses from erythema with dryness and cracking, through to more chronic changes with thickening and pigmentation. Dementia occurs late and is often preceded by apathy, depression and irritability.

Pellagra is now rare. Niacin is found in many foods and is added to breakfast cereals. Patients with severe malabsorptive states, food faddists and chronic alcoholics who do not eat are at risk of developing niacin deficiency. Pyridoxine is needed for the synthesis of nicotinamide and pyridoxine deficiency can therefore also cause pellagra.

Vitamin B_{12} deficiency is rarely caused by inadequate intake except among vegans. It causes a macrocytic anaemia, glossitis and, most importantly, neurological changes. If left untreated, subacute combined degeneration of the spinal cord can occur.

Deficiency of vitamin C, which is present in fresh fruit and vegetables, initially causes non-specific symptoms. Corkscrew hairs, swollen gums, perifollicular haemorrhages, bruising and anaemia are corrected with ascorbic acid supplementation and resumption of a normal diet.

Thiamine deficiency in the UK is almost exclusively seen in alcoholics and normally presents as Wernicke's encephalopathy. Ataxia, nystagmus, ophthalmoplegia and confusion are the classic findings and need treating promptly if a permanent dementia is to be prevented. Wet beriberi, causing oedema, and dry beriberi, presenting with a polyneuropathy, tend not to be seen outside South-East Asia.

Riboflavin deficiency has a less clearly defined deficiency syndrome: angular stomatitis, glossitis and dermatitis may occur.

Case 34

1   **B**   *Necator americanus*
    H   *Schistosoma mansoni*

He has two pathological processes: an acute bleed related to varices and therefore portal hypertension; and microcytosis with small, but visible, worms in the duodenum. His anaemia is likely to be due to the latter as he is unlikely to have had time to haemodilute from his bleed. The commonest cause of iron deficiency anaemia worldwide is hookworm infection (*Necator americanus* and *Ancylostoma duodenale*) which affects about 25% of the population. This is treatable with mebendazole.

Strongyloides stercoralis are not visible to the naked eye and cause malabsorption; *Ascaris lumbricoides* (roundworms) are much larger, mobile worms that cause pain and nausea; *Enterobius vermicularis* (threadworms) live in the colon, are more common in temperate climates and cause pruritus ani; and *Trichuris trichiura* (whipworm) infest the distal ileum and colon, causing, with heavy infestation, diarrhoea and bleeding.

He also has portal hypertension with completely normal liver function. Although it is possible to have cirrhosis due to viral hepatitis with normal liver function (about 5%), values tend towards the upper range of normal. Hence, another cause needs to be considered. *Schistosoma haematobium* infection can cause periportal fibrosis and portal hypertension with preserved hepatocellular function. *S. haematobium* affects the urinary tract. Treatment is with praziquantel and the standard management of portal hypertension.

Case 35

1   **B**   Angio-oedema of the bowel

The X-ray shows small-bowel obstruction, hence making Ogilvie's syndrome (chronic idiopathic intestinal pseudo-obstruction) unlikely: this normally presents with small- and large-bowel obstruction and has a less acute onset. Likewise, irritable bowel syndrome will not cause signs of a mechanical obstruction.

Adhesions are rarely a cause of obstruction in patients without a history of previous surgery. Rarely, idiopathic fibrous bands are seen at laparotomy for small-bowel obstruction.

Large gallstones can erode from the gallbladder directly into the small bowel, forming a fistulous connection. Subsequent obstruction can occur, caused by impaction of the gallstone, most commonly at the ileocaecal valve, but rarely at other points in the small bowel. Occasionally such stones are visible on X-rays but more commonly they are not. The classic sign of air in the biliary tree can help with the diagnosis although other causes of this sign, such as previous endoscopic sphincterotomy, must be remembered. In the case described there is no history suggestive of gallstone disease, nor are there any radiological signs to suggest this diagnosis.

Angio-oedema is a rare but recognised cause of small-bowel obstruction. Hereditary forms of the disease, due to a deficiency of C1 esterase inhibitor, are likely to present earlier in life and are usually associated with a family history. The clue in this case is the recent history of ACE inhibitor usage, which is the drug most commonly implicated in patients with non-hereditary angio-oedema. Symptoms can occur a matter of minutes, or many years after starting drug treatment, but normally occur within a few weeks of starting, or taking an increased dose of, ACE inhibitors. The symptoms are related to low levels of angiotensin II and a consequent increase in bradykinins. Alternative drugs should be used to prevent recurrence, or potentially lethal airway complications.

Case 36

1   **D**   Primary biliary cirrhosis

He is most likely to have primary biliary cirrhosis (PBC). This disease, of unknown aetiology, causes destruction of the small and medium-sized bile ducts. It tends to affect women more than men (9:1), between the ages of 30 and 60, although it can present outside these ages. Presenting features are fairly non-specific, fatigue and pruritus being the most common complaints. Abdominal pain is less frequently encountered. In the later stages of the disease, cirrhosis and its accompanying features may be found along with xanthelasmata, although examination early in the disease process may be normal.

Investigation shows marked elevation of the ALP and GGT with lesser increases in the transaminases. Serum immunoglobulins, particularly IgM, are also often elevated. Positive anti-mitochondrial (M2) antibodies have a sensitivity and specificity of over 90%. Biopsy allows confirmation of the diagnosis along with disease staging.

Treatment of pruritus is often difficult: colestyramine is the best treatment although it is often poorly tolerated, and antihistamines, opiate antagonists and rifampicin have a role to play. Ursodeoxycholic acid produces slight improvement in the time to transplantation and is the only effective treatment. Rising bilirubin levels indicate the need to consider transplantation, which may also be the only effective treatment for pruritus.

The history does not fit with either pancreatic carcinoma or gallstones, and haemochromatosis tends to cause a hepatitic rather than a cholestatic picture. The elevated IgM and HDL cholesterol levels are highly suggestive of PBC rather than of PSC.

Case 37

1   E   Boerhaave syndrome

Boerhaave syndrome, described by Herman Boerhaave in the 18th century, is spontaneous (as opposed to iatrogenic) oesophageal rupture. It is normally associated with violent vomiting and is more common in men than in women. It typically occurs in late middle age although it has been described in all age groups. Most commonly it occurs in the distal oesophagus, typically involving the left posterior wall.

Unlike in Mallory–Weiss syndrome, in which a partial-thickness tear occurs, haematemesis is uncommon in Boerhaave syndrome. Instead, the classic presentation is of vomiting with sudden onset of severe lower chest and upper abdominal pain. Other symptoms include shortness of breath, odynophagia and pleuritic pain. Findings include surgical emphysema (in about two-thirds of patients), pleural effusions (commonly left-sided) and, depending on the interval to presentation, features of mediastinitis. Chest X-rays can confirm pneumoperitoneum, pneumothorax, subcutaneous emphysema or pleural effusions, but, particularly early in the disease process, can be normal. Water-soluble contrast swallow is normally diagnostic; gastroscopy should be avoided to prevent worsening of the defect.

Management should be in conjunction with cardiothoracic surgeons as surgical intervention is often required.

Case 38

1   **D**   Carcinoid syndrome

Carcinoid syndrome develops when hepatic metastases occur from a carcinoid tumour. Men and women are equally affected and presentation tends to occur between the ages of 50 and 75. Carcinoid tumours are found most commonly in the ileum and appendix but can be located in many other places, both within and outwith the intestinal tract. Only a third of tumours are said to metastasise and, consequently, many are asymptomatic.

Carcinoids secrete many vasoactive molecules, including serotonin, which, in the absence of hepatic involvement, are metabolised in the liver. However, once secretion into the systemic circulation occurs, symptoms develop. Of these, debilitating diarrhoea, often associated with abdominal pain, is the most common. Flushing, which commonly affects the neck and face, may be associated with wheezing, and telangiectases may result. Alcohol and food intolerances, and exacerbation of symptoms by stress and some drugs, are not uncommon. The classic cardiac findings are of right-sided heart disease, namely tricuspid incompetence or pulmonary stenosis. Examination normally reveals hepatomegaly; imaging of the liver shows metastatic disease. Urinary levels of 5-hydroxyindoleacetic acid (5-HIAA) are normally increased. Treatment with octreotide, a somatostatin analogue, can improve symptoms and chemotherapy may be helpful in some patients.

Chronic pancreatitis tends to cause upper abdominal pain and malabsorptive, as opposed to watery, diarrhoea. Complications of coeliac disease are rare without a past history, although coeliac disease can be subclinical. Neither of these conditions, nor villous adenomas of the rectum are likely to have the associated symptoms described above.

IPSID is a proximal small-bowel lymphoproliferative condition that tends to present with malabsorption and weight loss. As with coeliac disease, it can progress to lymphoma.

Case 39

1 **B** Drug-related haemolysis
   C Iron deficiency due to malabsorption

The rash is dermatitis herpetiformis, which is an intensely itchy blistering
condition typically affecting the elbows, scalp, extensor surfaces of the
forearms and the buttocks. It is more common in males and can occur at
any age, although it tends to present in young adulthood. It is normally, if
not exclusively, associated with gluten-sensitive enteropathy. Treatment
of dermatitis herpetiformis includes strict adherence to a gluten-free diet.
Dapsone may be effective in controlling the rash but is often associated
with a mild, dose-related haemolytic anaemia. Haemolysis can,
however, be dramatic in patients with G6PD deficiency. Monitoring of
liver function tests and full blood counts is advised as dapsone can also
rarely cause liver dysfunction and aplastic anaemia. Drug treatment can
often be withdrawn after a period of adherence to a gluten-free
diet.
   Coeliac disease not infrequently presents with iron deficiency
anaemia and may also be complicated by folate deficiency. B_{12}
deficiency, in contrast, is less common as it is absorbed in the terminal
ileum. Hypocalcaemia occurs due to malabsorption of calcium and
vitamin D.

Case 40

1 **B** Hereditary non-polyposis colorectal cancer (HNPCC)

There is clearly a family cancer syndrome, making sporadic colorectal
carcinoma unlikely.

FAP is discussed elsewhere (pp. 190; 202). Attenuated FAP is associated
with different mutations in the *APC* gene and presents with a less severe
phenotype with fewer polyps than 'full-blown' FAP. Due to the fact that
FAP is a completely penetrant disorder, the family history presented here
cannot be explained by a diagnosis of FAP. Moreover, FAP is not
associated with gynaecological malignancy.

HNPCC is also an autosomal dominant disorder, the mutation being in a
DNA mismatch repair gene. HNPCC is defined as:

- Three or more family members affected by colorectal carcinoma (CRC)
  or
- Two or more with CRC and one with endometrial carcinoma:
      in two or more generations and
      one must be 50 years or under at diagnosis of malignancy and
      one of the relatives must be a first-degree relative of the other two
          (in this example, Case I.1).

Such a definition does not pick up all families with HNPCC but helps to focus on families with mismatch repair gene mutations. HNPCC predisposes to upper and lower gastrointestinal cancers, endometrial, ovarian and, less commonly, other cancers. As the name implies, patients with HNPCC tend to have fewer polyps than those with either FAP or Peutz–Jegher syndrome (see, p. 92); however, that is not to say that they do not get any polyps.

Patients with HNPCC are screened with colonoscopy from the age of 25, or 5 years earlier than the youngest age of diagnosis of colorectal cancer in the family. Screening for extra-intestinal cancer is also recommended by some centres.

Case 41

1   **B**   Endoscopic removal of the object

Ingested foreign objects are most commonly encountered in patients at the extremes of age. Most objects will pass through the gastrointestinal tract without complication. However, intervention is indicated in several instances as outlined below.

High-grade oesophageal obstruction, which presents with an inability to swallow even saliva, is an indication for intervention. High-risk objects impacted in the oesophagus, such as disk batteries or sharp objects, should be removed. Other objects should not be allowed to remain in the oesophagus for more than 24 hours.

Long objects that are unlikely to negotiate the duodenum often require endoscopic removal, as do large objects that will not progress beyond the pylorus. In the absence of symptoms, the latter can be monitored to see if they leave the stomach for several weeks before considering removal.

Objects that have already progressed beyond the duodenum can normally be monitored with weekly X-rays, surgical intervention being prompted by the object being stationary for over a week or by the onset of symptoms.

Once in the stomach (as in this case), sharp objects normally pass through the gastrointestinal tract safely. A small proportion, however, cause perforation and sharp objects within the stomach and proximal duodenum should therefore be carefully removed endoscopically. Otherwise, daily X-rays should be used to monitor the progress of more distal objects; surgery should be considered for objects that do not move for 72 hours and in patients in whom symptoms develop.

Narcotic packages should probably not be removed endoscopically in case of accidental rupture.

Chapter Four   Answers

PSYCHIATRY

Case 1

1   **H**   Delirium tremens

2   **D**   Pellagra

3   **A**   Pabrinex®

Pellagra is caused by nicotinic acid deficiency. It is characterised by the classical triad of:

- Dermatitis
- Diarrhoea
- Dementia.

Since the fortification of flour it has virtually disappeared in developed countries, except in association with chronic alcoholism and in a few case reports of the grossly malnourished homeless with only moderate alcohol consumption.

In their classic 1981 paper Ishii & Nishihara[1] showed that pellagra may be prevalent in this group even when the typical skin changes of pellagra (Casal's necklace) are not seen. This reinforces the importance of high-dose parenteral or intramuscular B vitamin therapy in all patients suspected of alcohol abuse or dependency.

Thiamine (vitamin B_1) deficiency is the better-known remediable vitamin deficiency frequently seen in this patient population. It leads to Wernicke–Korsakoff syndrome and irreversible brain damage if untreated.

According to Ishii & Nishihara:

- 20 of 74 cases of chronic alcoholism are found to have neuropathologically diagnosed pellagra at autopsy
- Admission diagnosis – delirium tremens 19/20
- Dementia–neuropsychiatric symptoms:
      confusion 20/20
      hallucinations 18/19
      insomnia 16/17
      tremor 14/17
      gait disturbance 19/20
      extrapyramidal rigidity of the limbs 16/17
      incontinence of urine and faeces 19/20

213

polyneuropathy 7/16
seizures 3/20
anxiety and depression in one-third to two-thirds
increased reflexes, especially in the lower limbs, seen in most cases,
    progressing to a paraparesis in a few
- Diarrhoea–gastrointestinal symptoms:
anorexia 12/20
diarrhoea 9/20
vomiting 5/20
constipation 3/20
glossitis 13/20
- Dermatitis–skin lesions 6/20:
vesicles or bullae on extremities
eczema-like lesions around the mouth and nose
desquamation and roughened skin over the hands
reddish discoloration scrotum
(none typical of pellagrous dermatitis).

Wernicke's encephalopathy is characterised by the triad of ataxia, confusion and ophthalmoplegia. Ocular motor abnormalities include horizontal nystagmus on lateral gaze, lateral rectus palsy (usually bilateral), conjugate gaze abnormalities and, rarely, ptosis. The complete triad, however, is seen in less than a third of cases. While hallucinations may be part of an acute confusional state, persecutory delusions are not commonly seen. Extrapyramidal rigidity is not seen and gastrointestinal symptoms are not part of the condition. Korsakoff's syndrome is often the permanent aftermath of Wernicke's encephalopathy and is associated with a marked anterograde memory impairment and confabulation.

[1] Ishii, N. and Nishihara, Y., Pellagra among chronic alcoholics: Clinical and pathological study of 20 necropsy cases. *Journal of Neurology*, Neurosurgery and psychiatry, 1981; 44: 209–215.

Case 2

1 **C** Toxicology screen
     D Urinary porphyrins

2 **E** Acute intermittent porphyria

Three common subtypes of porphyria give rise to neuropsychiatric disorders:

- Acute intermittent porphyria
- Variegate porphyria
- Coproporphyria.

The second two also cause cutaneous symptoms. Acute intermittent porphyria is the most common porphyria in European populations.

Acute attacks are characterised by the triad of: abdominal pain, neuropsychiatric symptoms and peripheral neuropathy. Abdominal pain is almost invariably present and believed to be due to an autonomic neuropathy. Vomiting, constipation, hypertension and tachycardia are also commonly seen. Peripheral neuropathy is predominantly motor, though sensory involvement may also occur and can mimic Guillain–Barré syndrome. The presence of central nervous system symptoms and abdominal pain in this case, however, make this diagnosis unlikely. Muscle weakness usually begins in the proximal muscles and typically affects the arms more commonly than the legs. Psychiatric manifestations are commonly seen and occasionally can completely dominate the clinical picture. Emotional disturbance is common and usually presents with acute depression or anxiety, though hypomania or even frank mania may also be seen. Lability of mood is also common. Clouding of consciousness may progress to an acute confusional state with auditory and visual hallucinations and delusions. Occasionally, schizophrenic symptoms such as social withdrawal, persecutory delusions and catatonia may also occur.

Drugs and the menstrual cycle are the most common precipitants of an attack, though alcohol, fasting, stress and infection have also been implicated. The occurrence of monthly luteal-phase attacks in women may lead to the false diagnoses of pre-menstrual tension or cycloid psychosis. Many of the drugs commonly used to treat the psychiatric manifestations are also implicated in triggering attacks, so extreme care must be taken in the management of these symptoms. Chlorpromazine is still considered the antipsychotic of choice, with limited experience with the newer atypical antipsychotics described. The tricyclic antidepressants as well as the SSRI fluvoxamine are contraindicated, though other SSRIs are probably safe. There are currently few data on the use of the newer combined action antidepressants such as venlafaxine and mirtazapine. For a full list of contraindicated drugs see the BNF[1].

Increased urinary excretion of porphobilinogen confirms the diagnosis of the acute attack. Screening tests using Ehrlich's reagent have been criticised because they lack sensitivity and should be confirmed by specific, quantitative assays. Porphobilinogen excretion may fall below the limits of detection rapidly after the onset of symptoms and a negative test should not rule out the diagnosis. In this instance, and if variegate porphyria is suspected, faecal and plasma porphyrins should be measured.

MDMA toxicity is associated with appetite suppression, nausea, muscle aches, trismus and bruxism. Insomnia can occur, as can tachycardia and hypertension and all usually resolve within 48 hours. The more serious complications include convulsions, rhabdomyolysis, DIC and acute renal failure associated with hyperpyrexia and dehydration. Psychiatric complications are diverse, including: panic; dysphoria, lasting 2–3 days; paranoia; auditory and complex visual hallucinations; morbid jealousy; and paranoid psychosis. This presentation would be compatible with a diagnosis of MDMA toxicity as would the hyponatraemia, though the peripheral neuropathy and abdominal symptoms point more to a diagnosis of AIP. Toxicology should be performed to rule out illicit drug use.

[1] http://www.bnf.org/bnf/bnf/current/openat/index.htm

Case 3

1   **D**   Neuroleptic malignant syndrome (NMS)

2   **D**   Creatine kinase

3   **C**   Dantrolene
     F   Bromocriptine

NMS is a rare but potentially life-threatening adverse effect of **all** anti-psychotics. It may occur at any time during the course of treatment though it is most commonly seen at the initiation of treatment or following rapid dose increases or reductions.

Diagnosis (according to DSM-4 Research Criteria[1]):

1   The development of severe muscle rigidity and elevated temperature associated with the use of neuroleptic medication.

2   Two (or more) of the following:
     • diaphoresis (sweating)
     • dysphagia
     • tremor
     • incontinence
     • changes in level of consciousness ranging from confusion to coma
     • mutism
     • tachycardia
     • elevated or labile blood pressure
     • leucocytosis
     • laboratory evidence of muscle injury (raised creatine kinase).

3   The symptoms in (1) and (2) are not due to another substance (eg phencyclidine) or a neurological or other general medical condition.

4   The symptoms in (1) and (2) are not better accounted for by a mental

disorder (eg mood disorder with catatonic features).[1]

Treatment:

Supportive – intravascular fluids, oxygen as required, close monitoring of temperature, pulse and BP. Stop the antipsychotic. Dantrolene reduces muscle tone by decreasing the release of calcium from the sarcoplasmic reticulum. Bromocriptine and amantadine have direct dopamine agonist properties and may be used to overcome the dopamine receptor blockade associated with antipsychotics.

[1] Taken from: American Psychiatric Association. *Diagnostic and Statistical Manual of Mental Disorders*, 4th edn.

Case 4

1   **B**   Serotonin syndrome

Serotonin syndrome is triggered by increased serotonergic stimulation. It typically results from pharmacodynamic and/or pharmacokinetic interactions between drugs that increase serotonergic activity. Its recognition followed the development of drugs that selectively enhance the activity if the serotonergic system. Increasing prescriptions for SSRIs and their potential interaction with medications with serotonergic activity used for other conditions have raised the importance of its recognition.

Mild symptoms such as restlessness, diaphoresis, tremor and shivering usually resolve rapidly on withdrawing the causative medication. Small doses of lorazepam may help to alleviate symptoms. Failure to recognise the development of serotonin syndrome may lead to the rapid development of more serious symptoms, such as myoclonus, confusion, hyperthermia convulsions, DIC, rhabdomyolysis and renal failure necessitating management in an ITU setting. Fatalities are described.

The most frequently associated drugs are combinations of SSRIs and monoamine oxidase inhibitors, including the newer reversible MAO-A inhibitors such as moclobemide and the MAO-B inhibitor selegiline used in the management of Parkinson's disease. It has also been described in combinations of SSRIs with tramadol, an analgesic with serotonin reuptake properties. There is also a risk when the triptans commonly used for migraine are combined with MAOIs (see list overleaf).

The symptoms of serotonin syndrome can be divided into: autonomic, neuromotor and cognitive-behavioural (see below).

Autonomic – diaphoresis, hyperthermia, hypertension, tachycardia, pupillary dilatation, nausea, diarrhoea, shivering.

Neuromotor – hyper-reflexia, myoclonus, restlessness, tremor, inco-ordination, rigidity, clonus, teeth chattering, trismus, seizures.

Cognitive/behavioural – confusion, agitation, anxiety, hypomania, insomnia, hallucinations, headache.

Behavioural –

	Clinical	Bloods	Cause
Serotonin syndrome	Typically rapid onset with hyper-reflexia, tremors, myoclonus, diaphoresis, confusion, agitation or shivering; muscular rigidity is not always present	Non-specific	Increased serotonergic tone
Neuroleptic malignant syndrome	Variable rapidity of onset; severe muscular rigidity, diaphoresis, delirium, fluctuating blood pressure, tachycardia, extrapyramidal symptoms	Elevated CPK, leucocytosis	Blockade of dopamine receptors or abrupt withdrawal of a dopamine agonist

Drugs associated with serotonin syndrome:

- Serotonin reuptake inhibitors – fluoxetine, sertraline, citalopram, escitalopram, paroxetine, clomipramine, venlafaxine, fluvoxamine, tramadol, trazodone, nefazodone, tricyclic antidepressants, amphetamine, cocaine, St John's wort
- Increased serotonin synthesis – tryptophan
- Inhibitors of serotonin metabolism – phenelzine, tranylcypromine, isocarboxazid, selegiline, moclobemide
- Increase serotonin release – MDMA (Ecstasy), amphetamine, cocaine, fenfluramine
- Increased serotonin activity – lithium, ECT
- Serotonin receptor agonists – buspirone, sumatriptan and other triptans (migraine).

Chapter Five   Answers

RENAL MEDICINE

Case 1

1   **C**   Indinavir

2   **C**   Urine for crystals

Drugs used in patients with HIV may cause acute renal failure (ARF). This occurs most commonly with protease inhibitors, in particular indinavir, by causing intratubular crystal obstruction. It has also been reported with ritonavir. Atorvastatin may cause myositis but in this patient the serum creatine kinase is normal.

Trimethoprin-sulfamethoxazole may cause acute interstitial nephritis presenting with ARF but the patient has been on this drug for a while with no problems.

Case 2

1   **C**   HIV-associated nephropathy (HIVAN)

HIV-associated nephropathy is associated with massive proteinuria, microscopic haematuria and renal failure, and predominantly occurs in black patients with HIV infection. In the era prior to combination antiretroviral therapy, this led to rapid progression to end-stage renal failure. The classic lesion on renal histology is the collapsing variant of secondary focal segmental glomerulosclerosis. The histological features may also represent heroin associated nephropathy.

Schistosoma haematobium infection of the lower urinary tract is associated with ureteral strictures and bladder cancer. It may cause an immune complex-mediated mesangial glomerulonephritis.

Case 3

1   **E**   Anti-glomerular basement membrane disease

Initial presentation was of a patient with subclinical lung haemorrhage and acute renal failure. Often, lung haemorrhage may present without haemoptysis and in this case was incorrectly diagnosed as a chest infection. The clinical presentation and subsequent progress is consistent with the syndrome of alveolar haemorrhage and renal failure caused by anti-glomerular basement membrane (GBM) antibodies (Goodpasture's syndrome). Other causes of this syndrome are Wegener's granulomatosis (ANCA-positive in 95% of patients), SLE, Churg–Strauss syndrome and mixed essential cryoglobulinaemia. Microscopic polyangiitis may also cause this syndrome, but only up to 10% of patients are ANCA-negative. Goodpasture's syndrome is rare and presents with lung haemorrhage and/or rapidly progressive glomerulonephritis. Diagnosis is made by the presence of circulating anti-GBM antibodies and on renal biopsy. Typical appearances are of diffuse proliferative glomerulonephritis with variable degrees of necrosis, crescent formation, glomerulosclerosis and tubular loss. Treatment is with cytotoxic immunosuppression and plasma exchange. Poor prognostic factors are advanced renal failure on presentation and the degree of crescent formation.

Case 4

1   **A**   Anti-glomerular basement membrane disease

Alport's is an inherited disorder resulting in microscopic haematuria, progressive nephritis with renal impairment, sensorineural deafness and ocular abnormalities. It is due to mutations of tissue-specific type IV collagen chains, leading to formation of autoantibodies similar to those in Goodpasture's syndrome. Therefore, a minority of Alport's patients with a renal transplant develop a rapidly progressive glomerulonephritis indistinguishable from Goodpasture's syndrome but without pulmonary haemorrhage. Treatment is similar to that of *de novo* anti-GBM disease but treatment efficacy is limited.

Opportunistic infections are common in transplant recipients, especially with over-immunosuppression. Common infections include cytomegalovirus, varicella zoster virus and fungal diseases. Post-transplant lymphoproliferative disorder is an uncommon but serious manifestation, the majority of which are of B-cell clonality associated with Epstein–Barr virus. Treatment is often by a reduction of the immunosuppression and chemotherapy. Graft loss is common.

Case 5

1   **B**   Infective endocarditis

The history and investigations are consistent with infective endocarditis. One third of patients with bacterial endocarditis develop ARF. The glomerulonephritis is associated with desposition of immune complexes containing bacterial antigens in glomeruli. Cryoglobulins (polyclonal or type III) are present in 50% of subjects.

HIVAN occurs almost exclusively in black patients, and they tend to be normotensive. Microscopic polyangiitis may present with nail-fold vasculitic lesions but these patients are commonly ANCA-positive. Renal TB is associated with an insidious onset of renal impairment with asymptomatic urinary abnormalities such as persistent sterile pyuria. It may or may not be associated with extrarenal systemic manifestations.

Case 6

1   **D**   von Hippel–Lindau disease

Von Hippel–Lindau disease is an autosomal dominant condition that manifests in CNS haemangioblastomas, renal and pancreatic cysts, renal carcinoma and phaeochromocytomas. Renal cysts are usually multiple and bilateral and are often associated with solid tumours. Other causes of renal cystic disease include ADPKD, ARPKD, tuberose sclerosis complex, medullary cystic disease and renal cystic dysplasia.

ADPKD commonly presents in adulthood and may be associated with intracranial berry aneurysms. ARPKD commonly presents in either the neonatal period or up to adolescence with renal impairment. In TSC 80% of affected individuals have seizures and manifest with angiomyolipomas in skin and visceral organs.

Case 7

1   **B**   cANCA-positive vasculitis

This is a classic presentation of Wegener's granulomatosis. It is a necrotising granulomatous vasculitis affecting the small vessels, associated with circulating anti-neutrophil cytoplasmic antibodies (ANCA). It may manifest in a combination of upper and/or lower respiratory tract and/or renal disease. On immunofluorescence, ANCA staining is cytoplasmic with specificity to proteinase-3. pANCA-positive vasculitis and HSP are not classically associated with upper respiratory tract symptoms. Lupus nephritis is associated with a positive ANA and hypocomplementaemia.

Case 8

1   **E**   Membranous nephropathy

Nephrotic syndrome with hepatitis B infection and carriage is associated with secondary membranous nephropathy. Other common causes of secondary membranous nephropathy include SLE, drugs (gold, penicillamine) and malignancies.

The duration of diabetes and the absence of other microvascular complications such as retinopathy make diabetic nephropathy less likely. Renal TB is not commonly associated with nephrotic syndrome. MCGN is a rare cause in a hepatitis B-positive patient and is typically associated with red cell casts.

Case 9

1   D   Diabetic glomerulosclerosis

The duration of poorly controlled diabetes and evidence of microvascular disease make diabetic nephropathy the most likely diagnosis. The biopsy shows mesangial expansion with a Kimmelstiel–Wilson nodule at the top of the glomerulus, typical of diabetic glomerulosclerosis. The incidence of membranous nephropathy and of minimal-change disease is increased in diabetics compared with non-diabetic patients but on light microscopy the glomeruli will show capillary loop thickening and normal architecture respectively.

Case 10

1   C   Henoch–Schönlein purpura

In a young patient with microscopic haematuria and renal impairment, the differential diagnosis includes IgA nephropathy and thin-membrane disease. Both IgA nephropathy (IgAN) and Henoch–Schönlein nephritis are characterised by mesangial IgA deposition. The latter is differentiated from IgAN by extrarenal manifestations, such as purpura (as in this gentleman), polyarthralgia, and abdominal pain caused by gut vasculitis with IgA deposition. HSP is uncommon after the second decade of life and the renal involvement is often transient. The rash is a purpuric vasculitis, usually spreading on the extensor surfaces. Histology shows a leucocytoclastic vasculitis with IgA deposits in blood vessel walls.

Case 11

1   A   Primary hyperoxaluria

Elevated urinary oxalate levels may be due to increased dietary intake, malabsorption or an inherited enzyme deficiency that leads to excessive metabolism of oxalate (primary hyperoxaluria). There are three types: types I and III are due to an enzyme defect in the liver glyoxalate pathway and in type II there is failure of reduction of glyoxalate to glycolate. Type I is the commonest and results in widespread calcium oxalate deposition throughout the body.

Treatment of primary hyperoxaluria is aimed at increasing urinary pH to make calcium oxalate more soluble. This is by administering supplemental citrate and magnesium. Renal insufficiency is common and patients require a combined liver and kidney transplant in type I disease.

Her normal serum calcium and phosphate levels are not consistent with hyperparathyroidism.

Diabetes insipidus is characterised by polyuria and polydipsia. The acquired form may be due to electrolyte abnormalities (hypokalaemia, hypercalcaemia), chronic renal failure or lithium therapy. Nephrocalcinosis is uncommon.

Case 12

1   **D**   Intravenous fresh frozen plasma

Acute renal failure, anaemia and thrombocytopenia with fragmented red cells are diagnostic of haemolytic uraemic syndrome in the absence of neurological signs. It is commonly associated with a diarrhoeal illness. Treatment is supportive. The first-line therapy is infusion of fresh frozen plasma or plasma exchange, the latter especially if there is neurological involvement or if the patient is oligo-anuric. Treatment efficacy can be monitored by measurement of plasma LDH. Haemodialysis is only indicated if the patient is oligo-anuric and is not responding to specific treatment. There is no known role for tranexamic acid or vitamin K.

Case 13

1   **C**   Analgesic nephropathy

The patient in question has chronic renal failure due to the long-term use of non-steroidal anti-inflammatory drugs (NSAIDS). There is no clue in the history that he has been taking over-the-counter herbal medications. The duration of diabetes mellitus and the normal blood pressure with no evidence of other end-organ damage (normal fundi, no LVH on voltage criteria in the ECG) exclude both diabetic nephropathy and hypertensive nephrosclerosis. As he is on ACE inhibitors, the absence of bruits and symmetrical kidneys make renovascular disease unlikely.

Chronic NSAID abuse leads to renal injury due to renal papillary necrosis and chronic interstitial nephritis. The degree of renal injury correlates with the duration of use and analgesic load. There is no specific treatment apart form avoidance of NSAIDs.

Some Chinese herbs have been implicated in the development of rapidly progressive renal failure due to interstitial nephritis and progressive tubulo-interstitial fibrosis.

Case 14

1   **D**   Pure red cell aplasia

Pure red cell aplasia (PRCA) is a rare condition defined by the absence of erythroblasts in the bone marrow, leading to profound anaemia with normal leucocyte and platelet counts, and characterised by low or absent circulating reticulocytes. Serum iron and ferritin rise sharply as iron cannot be incorporated into the erythrocytes.

PRCA occurs due to neutralising antibodies to erythropoietin. There has been a recent increase in PRCA in patients with chronic kidney disease on subcutaneous erythropoietin alpha. Treatment includes discontinuation of the EPO preparation and repeated transfusions.

The normal MCV and WCC make hypothyroidism and chronic lymphocytic leukaemia unlikely.

In myelofibrosis the blood film shows a leucoerythroblastic picture with an increased reticulocyte count.

Case 15

1   **A**   Oral ferrous sulphate

Anaemia is almost universal in patients with chronic kidney disease; it is characteristically normochromic and normocytic and is associated with erythropoietin (Epo) deficiency and shortening of red cell survival. Eventually, patients are commenced on erythropoietin. Iron stores should be optimised before beginning erythropoietin. The first step should be oral iron and if this does not normalise the serum ferritin, then a course of intravenous iron is used. Red cell transfusions should be avoided unless in an emergency, as this patient will develop circulating antibodies which would make future transplantation more difficult.